Hov

To A Diet

The Ultimate Guide To "Hacking" Your
Brain For Unstoppable Motivation
And Lifelong Diet Success

Derek Doepker

FREE GIFT

I'd like to reward you with **free** access to my premium fitness newsletter.

You'll learn my best cutting edge strategies for getting fit on a busy schedule, how to reprogram your genetics, and get "insider" tips picked up from the world's elite fitness trainers. Simply visit excuseproof.com and get free instant access to the Excuse Proof Fitness Survival Guide and newsletter today.

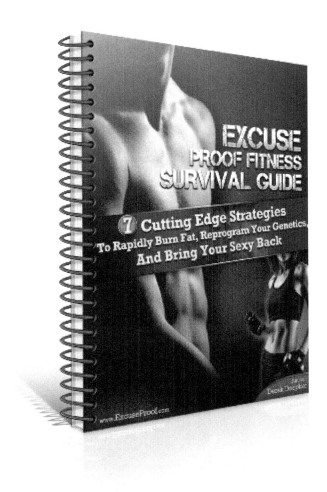

Disclaimer:

Table of Contents

Preface

Do you know why most dieting approaches are surefire ways to fail to get long term results with health and weight loss? And do you know what you can do instead?

Do you know there is a simple technique to practically "force" yourself to stick to a goal (regardless of willpower), and *enjoy* the process?

Do you know the 4 fundamental emotional needs that drive your behavior? For most people these needs are sabotaging their efforts to stick to a diet. If you know how to utilize these drives for good, you can get yourself motivated to achieve any change in your life you want!

Do you know there's a way to make enough delicious healthy meals to last for days with only 5-10 minutes of prep time in the kitchen?

Do you know that eating a whole foods diet can actually be cheaper than eating junk food and that a typical "junk food" diet can actually cost far more money?

I don't know about you, but I didn't any of these things when I first made the commitment to get myself in shape and start eating healthy.

I always assumed "dieting" or "eating healthy" was a miserable thing to be endured for the sake of better health or a better body. I forced myself to eat boring and bland foods that I hated. I forced myself to spend all my money on expensive health foods and to spend hours preparing meals with time that would have been much better spent elsewhere.

But all of that changed over the course of 8 years with extensive hours of research relating to nutrition, weight loss, and cooking combined with studying advanced cognitive psychology and adult behavioral psychology in order to bring this book to you. My intense years of study led to discovering some amazingly powerful mind "hacks" and lifestyle "hacks" that make sticking with a healthy diet so "stupid-simple," someone had to write a book about it.

"How To Stick To A Diet" is a result of that research, experimentation, and the collective wisdom of literally hundreds of experts in the fields of nutrition, health, fitness, and psychology.

This book is designed to show you how to work with your own psychology and life's circumstances (schedule, budget, taste in food) so YOU are in control of your food choices as opposed to your habits, addictions, cravings, finances, emotions, which can dictate how you eat.

For those whom believe that diets don't work, you'll find the reasons why this is both true <u>and</u> false. Following most conventional diet advice commonly leads to incredibly high rates of failure, but you're about to learn how to avoid all of those mistakes and get the fit body and ultimate health you desire.

The information found in this book will help you whether you follow a particular diet like Paleo, vegetarian, vegan, raw foods, low-carb, low-fat, Mediterranean, macrobiotic, etc. or whether you just simply want to make better food choices each day. Whether you're seeking better health, less fat, more muscle, or just desire to feel more in control of your life without the misery of "dieting," this book is designed to help you with your *your* personal goals.

As long as your approach is reasonable (not overly restrictive or unhealthy), you're going to learn how you can "rewrite" the programming in your brain to have unstoppable "stick-to-it-iveness," even if you currently feel you lack motivation or willpower.

How can this be done?

By sharing with you some of the very same cutting edge (and sometimes highly unconventional) strategies that have the power to transform your brain. There will also be plenty of practical everyday tips, tricks, and lifestyle strategies that have personally allowed me to maintain a lean six pack all year round with ease. Even better, all of this can be done without depriving yourself, without being miserable, and without spinning your wheels going from diet to diet never getting results.

These strategies worked even when I was a broke and busy college student with the pickiest taste in foods and an absolute feeling of disgust for any "health foods." But it's not my results that matter. The reason I'm sharing these techniques is because these strategies have also helped thousands successfully make a permanent shift into a healthier, leaner, and more fit body.

Just imagine how easy would it be to stick with a diet if you knew:

- Why following most diets will guarantee you'll never achieve *long-term* health and fitness. How by approaching diets the *right way*, you can achieve **permanent** success.

- Why most typical "goal setting" advice is incomplete, and how to use a "missing link" to ensure you will stick to your goals no matter what.

- Why most "get-fit-quick" schemes are not only ineffective, but can actually cause psychological harm!

- Why you may feel stressed out about the idea of dieting, and how you can free yourself of feeling overwhelmed when approaching diet or even other areas your life. TIP: Discover this secret, and your happiness will skyrocket regardless of your diet!

- How to strengthen your willpower and use it properly so you never feel overly stressed out or like you're having to constantly "force" yourself to stay on track.

- Why "cheating" on your diet may be exactly what you need to avoid plateus, and how to wrong type of cheating could spell absolute disaster! Understand this, and you'll be able to always "have your cake and eat it too!"

- How to turn every failure into a success and prevent them from making you feel like giving up.

- How to use an exercise to stick to your diet that is so powerful, a version of it was actually used to brainwash prisoners of war into agreeing with the enemy! Although this is perfectly safe, use this only if you are really serious about making a permanent change in your behavior.

- How to avoid feeling like a slave to your cravings by using a stupid simple language based "mind hack" that research has shown significantly curbs junk food cravings.

- Why sugar and salt cravings may *not* just be in your head, but could be the signs of an underlying deficiency that can easily be fixed with a trip to your local health food store.

- How "common sense" diet advice may be keeping you stuck spinning your wheels, and why breaking all of the rules can get you the healthy fit body you've been looking for.

- How to purchase organic quality food at <u>wholesale</u> prices so money never has to be an obstacle to achieving better health.

- How to get the highest quality protein shakes and supplements that cost as little as ¼ of retail store costs. Never pay too much for your supplements again.

- Why "not enough time" is *always* a lie, and how even the busiest people on the planet are able to stick with their diets no matter how crazy their lives are.

- And much, *much* more!

This book is NOT for...

1. *People who want someone telling them exactly how to eat and spewing out more "dogma" about the so called rules of healthy eating and dieting.*

This book is not about telling anyone what they should and shouldn't eat, although there will be plenty of resources provided for you to learn more about nutrition. Rather, it's about empowering you to make the choices that best suit your life and belief systems. So, if you need a diet book telling you what to eat or not eat, this isn't it. (Although there are some good tips and recipes) This book is meant to fill in the gaps with what most diet books leave out, and that is how to get a diet to work **with** your life rather than against it.

2. People looking for an "easy" fix and who want to avoid a challenge.

While many of the strategies in this book are simple, if someone goes into something believing it must be easy, they may not be willing to face the obstacles that will inevitably occur going through the process. The truth is, there are no easy buttons to making changes in your life because all change require effort.

The good news is, if you are willing to make a commitment to change yourself for the better and accept that it can be an exciting challenge, you may find it's far easier than you ever imagined it to be.

3. People who take diets and dieting too seriously.

Taking better care of your body and health is meant to be a part of your life, not the sole purpose of it. You will make mistakes, and I know this because everyone makes mistakes including myself. Rather than seeing a mistake as complete failure and an excuse to give up, it's better to accept that you'll make mistakes along the way right now and welcome those mistakes as learning opportunities. Making better choices about what you put into your bodies and perhaps getting leaner and sexier along the way can be achieved with these mindset techniques.

This book may not for those who want to argue about whether something is or isn't really "healthy." Even though I often use that word, it is admittedly extremely subjective and used mostly as a relative term to oppose "junk food" (another subjective term). Regardless of one's thoughts on what constitutes "healthy" or "junk," well over 90% of this book will be relevant.

4. People who are looking for the ultimate diet book.

This book is written by a person who has had real struggles with diets but has worked through them. I will "keep it real" with you.

This is not an "academic book" or a Wikipedia entry with countless citations. I've decided to use my research and real world experimentation to distill everything down into really simple guidelines for the everyday person to follow.

That being said, I do believe giving some in depth explanations are necessary. Please understand that when you can comprehend at least some of the reasons *why* certain things are recommended, it makes it far easier to apply the information for lasting results.

5. *People who are not willing to make a change.*

If you read this book and expect that simply seeing the words on the page will magically make you change, it won't happen. While there's plenty of inspiration here that may prompt you to a greater desire to take control of your health, I, and no one else, can *make* those changes for you.

If you think something sounds too unusual to work, then you're free to accept it or reject it. In fact, I encourage you not to blindly follow something just because a person wrote it in a book.

But ask yourself, is what I'm doing right now working? If not, doesn't that mean I need to try something different? Not everything in this book will work for everyone as we're all unique. I encourage you to experiment and give new things an honest effort to discover what is most effective for you.

Congratulations!

You've decided to take control of your health. You've already taken many of the most difficult steps in the journey of dieting and health by identifying your obstacles, seeking out reliable solutions, and then taking action to get and use the resources you need for success by getting this book.

You've already shown you're someone who will take action to overcome any obstacles we are challenged with everyday. You can successfully continue your healthy journey by applying the empowering techniques this book has to offer.

Who Are You And Why Should I Listen To You?

I didn't always use to be the super healthy and motivated guy I am today. I started out as a 17 year old high school student who ate fast food *every single* night. I refused to eat healthy. I never exercised leaving me one of the most out of shape guys in my class.

I started to read about the effects an unhealthy diet has on the body and made a commitment to change. Even though I hated eating healthy foods, I discovered how to change my mindset and stick with with a healthy eating plan that allowed me to add over 30 pounds of muscle in several months, and get a ripped six pack in the process.

I then went on to help my overweight friend, Shane Edele, drop from 220 pounds to 168 pounds. He now maintains a six pack year round. We've both been able to maintain our physiques and healthy eating habits with ease over the course of 8 years since we've started.

How did we manage to go from eating horrendous diets to doing a complete 180 and getting strong, lean, athletic bodies? And most importantly, how did we manage to make these healthier habits stick for years on end with no sign or temptation of ever going back to our old ways like some others do?

By following the valuable information and life changing techniques you're about to read, you'll discover how to successfully stick to your resolutions.

Today, I am a fitness expert and founder of Excuse Proof Fitness at excuseproof.com. I wrote this book because I want to help others avoid all of the mistakes I've made, and give you the secrets I've picked up over the years for how to make healthy decisions even when if you're on a budget, busy, and/or unmotivated.

Come check out my blog Excuse Proof Fitness at excuseproof.com, subscribe to my youtube channel at www.youtube.com/excuseproof, and I hope you'll come to know and trust me for keeping it real with you when it comes to fitness advice.

These techniques are based on what has worked for me and many others. You may find they are simply a spring board for your own growth patterns. Simply recognize these techniques here are useful tools that can be used in all aspects of your life, but they're not the only means of success. All any book or program can do is provide you with tools, but it is you and your actions that are ultimately the source of your results.

Here are a couple photos of myself to show you the results I've achieved.

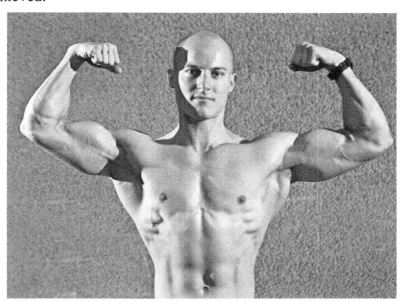

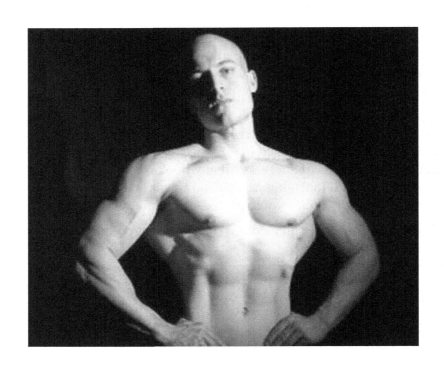

Why Do Diets Often Fail?

A startling statistic has shown that the majority of people who follow a calorie restricted diet approach and lose weight end up just as overweight or more so several years down the road. Some research has even shown those who have gone on diets may actually be more likely to be overweight down the road than those who didn't!

See:http://magazine.ucla.edu/exclusives/dieting_no-go/index1.html

While there's certainly many people who successfully lose weight and keep it off through a careful diet, and the true percentage of people who fail to achieve *long-term* success on a diet may not actually be as high as in the studies (due to issues with the way these studies are conducted), it is still pretty easy to dismiss diets and dieting as an ineffective approach for weight loss.

Whether the reasons for diets failing to get long-term weight loss results are physiological (fighting the body's fat "set-point") and/or psychological (no one wants to feel deprived of the foods they enjoy), "diets don't work" has become a common mantra.

I'm here to argue that the statement "diets don't work" is both true <u>and</u> false. The key is to understand is how language and context plays a role in all of this. You're about to find out how conventional thinking on diets can be sabotaging your results and keeping you stuck, and how one simple shift in thinking may be all it takes to finally achieve lasting success.

The first thing to realize is that "diet" can refer to a number of things. Looking at a dictionary definition (http://www.merriam-webster.com/dictionary/diet), we can see that diet can refer to either a means of eating sparingly to reduce weight OR it can be used to simply refer to the habitual way someone eats.

The problem is, for some people when they hear the word diet, they automatically assume it means a restricted way of eating. Typically along the lines of eating far less food than usual (starving yourself), and/or only eating boring and bland "health" food like plain lettuce, broccoli, and celery sticks.

This means that the word diet gets linked with feelings of agonizing restriction and deprivation of one of life's greatest pleasures, eating great tasting food. It's no wonder some people have such as hard time sticking with a diet when the idea of a diet feels like a prison sentence!

But I would say even if a person eats ice cream and cheeseburgers all day, they're still on a "diet." That is, we're all on a diet in that we all have a particular, often habitual way of eating. For some people, that's simply a "see food" diet of you see it, you eat it.

This leads me to another phrase I don't care for, and that is "going on a diet." To me, since a diet is something that everyone is already "on," it's impossible to go "on a diet." Rather, one can only "adjust their diet" or perhaps "go on a *specific* diet." This once again has to do with defining diet as "the way someone eats."

Here's another issue with "going on a diet," and that is the implication that if you "go on a diet" you may then "come off a diet." What good is it to actually find a great diet that will get you the healthy body you've always wanted, only to "come off" that diet, eat like crap, and then lose all the beneficial results you've achieved?

A person's diet for better or worse should be looked at as a way of life.

How Can One Simple Shift Help With Sticking To A Diet?

The very first step in sticking with a diet, is to not see a diet as a means to an end, but rather as an ongoing lifestyle **habit** that you are already engaged in.

Instead of looking at a diet as something to *add* into your life, see a diet as something you're already "on." When you look at it this way, "sticking with" a diet really means sticking with certain dietary **habits** you deem beneficial.

This means all you have to do is simply substitute a few dietary choices you're already making with a few better choices, and make these better choices your new "normal."

So now the question is this; "How is my current diet getting me closer to or further from the goals I have?"

Since there are countless books and resources out there for figuring out what to eat for any particular goal, and many people already have a basic idea of how they can start eating better, I won't include that in this book.

But once you know what you need to change, the next question (which this book will answer) is this: "How can I make these changes become my new regular dietary habit?"

This is a much needed "missing link" that most diet programs don't include. It doesn't help that many diets are simply designed to be "short term" fixes, and even the ones that are sustainable over the long term don't make the effort to show the users how to make it part of their lifestyle. While some short-term approaches certainly have their place, it's absolutely critical you understand how to control your dietary habits so you can sustain any benefits a better diet will give you for the rest of your life.

By reading the following pages, you're going to be let in on the secret for how to keep your healthy dietary habits for the rest of your life so you'll never have to worry about losing the amazingly fit and healthy body you've worked so hard for. And as a bonus, once you understand these secrets, you'll be able to apply these strategies to get yourself to stick to just about any habit you're looking to add into your life! How cool is that?

Why Is It So Hard To Get And Stay Motivated?

Whether it's sticking with a diet, quitting smoking, or staying on an exercise program, there's something inherently challenging about making a resolution and sticking with it no matter how motivated someone is to change.

This is in part because people often have a misconception about motivation. They think it is something that a person has or doesn't have to varying degrees, but in truth, everyone is *already* motivated.

Think about this, if a person sits around all day and watches TV instead of getting something else done that they'd like to do like go to the gym, that doesn't mean they're "unmotivated." It means they're *more* motivated to watch TV than go to the gym! If that person says, "yeah, well I want to go to the gym but I just don't have the energy," then they are more motivated to conserve energy than expend it.

But why does one thing "motivate" a person to do something while the same thing may not motivate another person to do it? Take health risks for instance. The health consequences of smoking may be enough to "motivate" one person to quit, but not another.

The reason something motivates one person and not another is that we all have different priorities, and our priorities are based on what we *perceive* will minimize pain and increase pleasure for us. Since we're usually not dealing with *physical* pain when it comes to our diets, that means this pleasure and pain is typically emotional/psychological in nature.

So what determines whether or not something will create emotional pain or pleasure? We can isolate a few core emotional wants/needs that are common to all human beings which drive, on the deepest level, all of our behavior.

(I use want/need and "drives" interchangeably to refer to the underlying emotional feelings that we all "crave" as human beings)

While different experts may have different classifications for these emotional wants, for the sake of this book we're going to cover these 4 wants that are the source of all your diet motivation:

1. **Security** (Survival, meeting basic physical needs, having enough money/resources, etc.)

2. **Control** (Feeling a sense of freedom, having choices, having a sense of certainty)

3. **Validation / Approval** (Feeling valued, fitting in, being accepted, wanting to contribute)

4. **Excitement** (Fun and entertainment, feeling like life has purpose, hope for a better future, wanting some <u>uncertainty</u> – note: wanting uncertainty *opposes our drive for wanting certainty, i.e. we have conflicting wants!*)

Even though we all have these same basic emotional wants/needs, the way we've been conditioned to fulfill these wants is unique to each person. The various beliefs each person has about how they can best satisfy their emotional wants is what leads to differing personalities despite the fact that we all have a similar underlying "human psychology."

Let's take a look at how these emotional wants play out in the "real world" with underlying thoughts and feelings a person may have when attempting to either improve their diet vs. keeping their dietary "status quo."

Validation As A Motivator To Keep Old Diet - Will I get laughed at by others for making healthier diet choices? Will I be able to fit in at parties or celebrations if I'm eating differently and can't enjoy all of the foods I'm offered? Will I offend my friends and family if I refuse to eat what they offer? Will those I'm close to not approve of me changing my diet?

Validation As A Motivator To Improve Diet – Are people laughing at me for my unhealthy diet or out of shape body? Will people like me more if I take better care of my body? Will I fit in more if I have a better looking body as a result of changing my diet?

Control As A Motivator To Keep Old Diet – Will following another diet make me feel deprived? Will I be unable to find ways to get the new foods I need? Will I be unable to do the things in my life I enjoy doing if I'm stuck trying to follow a new diet?

Control As A Motivator To Improve Diet – If I eat differently, will my energy levels improve allowing me to do more things I'd like to do? Will improving my diet make me feel like I'm more in control of my choices and improve my self-esteem? Will being more fit give me more options for what I can wear?

Security As A Motivator To Keep Old Diet – Will a new diet cost me a lot of time or money? Will a new diet be potentially unhealthy or harmful?

Security As A Motivator To Improve Diet – Will improving my diet prolong my life? Will improving my diet save money time or money?

Excitement As A Motivator To Keep Old Diet – Will a new diet be boring? Will a new diet taste bland? Will I no longer be able to enjoy my favorite foods and restaurants?

Excitement As A Motivator To Improve Diet – Will improving my diet give me the body and energy to pursue things I'm passionate about? Will a new diet expose me to new foods and flavors that I may love?

Notice how all of these example thoughts and feelings a person may have about diets aren't necessarily based on anything objectively true or false. It's all based on beliefs one has built up around what "dieting" means. Following a better diet could mean less freedom and greater pain to one person, while the *exact same* dietary changes may mean *more* freedom and greater pleasure to another person simply based on the psychological beliefs each person has.

We also build up layers and layers of beliefs around diets which creates conflicting drives of wanting to improve our diets while at the same time wanting to keep our dietary status quo.

To give an example, if someone believes that changing their diet is going to be time consuming, but on the other hand believes it will make them look and feel better because they're overweight, then they have two conflicting drives working against each other creating a "tug-of-war" effect. Part of them wants to save time as a matter of either fulfilling security, control, and/or excitement, while another part of them wants to look and feel better to fulfill a wanting for validation, security (protect their health), and/or control (able to do more things if more fit).

This person may face constant emotional turmoil of, on one hand, feeling like a miserable slave if they're sticking with a "weight loss" diet. Then on the other hand they feel guilt and embarrassment if they don't stick with this weight loss diet and stay out of shape. It's seems like a catch-22 that can't be solved.

To make matters worse, many times we aren't even aware of what is driving our behavior. Someone may think that they don't want to change their diet because it would be time consuming to prepare different meals, but their true motivation for not changing is that deep down inside they believe their friends will laugh at them for being a "health nut." This is all going on subconsciously without a person even knowing what's driving their behavior.

To put it simply, virtually *everything* you do, you do because you feel it benefits and meets one or more of these emotional wants. Therefore, if you're attempting to make any change in your life, you're going to have to recognize that you're basically telling your brain to give up something it feels is beneficial or even *essential* to your happiness and survival.

Now imagine how hard it would be for someone to change their diet if the only way they knew how to fulfill their wanting for excitement was through the foods they eat. If they then try to change to a boring and bland "health food" diet, and didn't do anything to spice up their new diet or meet their wanting for excitement through other means, they will either become completely miserable or they will eventually break down and go back to their old habits to fulfill that need for excitement again.

No wonder sticking to a diet, or making *any* change for that matter is so difficult! But, does it really need to be? The good news is when you understand this, and understand how to work *with* your psychology and emotions rather than against them, you can not only successfully make a lasting change, but find the process enjoyable and rewarding leading to even **greater** happiness.

So if you're ready, let's dive deeper into how we can utilize this knowledge to reprogram your mind for unstoppable motivation.

What Is The First Step In Making A Change?

We've established that the best way to approach a diet is to realize you're already on one and therefore you're simply working on changing *preexisting* behaviors/habits vs. doing something new all together. We've also established that you're already "motivated," but that someone may either be motivated in the wrong direction or have conflicting motivations.

Now we need to breakdown how we can apply this information to make a lasting change in not only your behavior, but how you actually feel *about* your behaviors. "Willpower" (which we'll cover in a bit) is necessary, but it is only one tool in making changes in your life. Without addressing your emotional wants, you'll always feel like you're fighting an uphill battle by just "forcing" yourself to do things.

The first step in making any change in your life is **awareness**.

Without awareness, you are simply like a robot running on autopilot following programmed routines and habits without much conscious thought.

A more everyday example of this would be driving in a car, and then not remembering the last few minutes of driving only to "snap back to reality" and realize that somehow or another, you've safely driven the past few miles without even being aware of it.

Or perhaps eating an entire tub of ice cream and then looking back and going, "Wow! How did that happen?"

All of these instances, from the more deep trances of driving and TV watching, to the more everyday decisions of what to eat result from the habitual way our brain works. Over 90% of our decisions are made without any conscious effort or deep understanding *why* we made those decisions in the moment. In essence, the feeling that you are always aware of your thoughts and rationalizations for making most of your decisions is an illusion.

By actually *practicing* awareness, you can start to notice your habitual thoughts, feelings, and underlying beliefs behind every action you take. This is actually more difficult than it sounds, but luckily for us we're mostly just focusing our practice of awareness around diet for the time being. As you get better, you can (and should) apply greater awareness of each moment to all areas of your life.

How Can I Apply Awareness To Change My Behavior?

Awareness is quite simply observing your thoughts and feelings *without judgment*. You become both a participant and observer of your life.

The biggest trick with awareness is that you're not actually trying to change your behaviors, thoughts, or feelings when you're observing them. A person may go ahead and eat an entire tub of ice cream, but they should notice all of their thoughts, feelings, and everything they are experiencing before, during, and after eating the ice cream.

While this may sound odd at first, consider that this person eating the ice cream may discover how they didn't want to eat the ice cream because they were *physically* hungry, but rather because they're experiencing an emotional emptiness inside. The ice cream was satisfying an emotional want, not a physical one.

Don't worry, I'm not going to get all "therapist" on you by talking about how you need to get in touch with your "inner child" or anything to simply start eating better. But realize this is an important step because knowing what is driving your behaviors and patterns in life will later allow you to make conscious choices as to whether you want to continue in those behaviors, or make changes to them.

A "warm-up" exercise to get better at awareness is to just start to be aware of your right hand, or any part of your body for a couple minutes. Put your mind into that body part and just notice all the feelings and sensations in that body part. Feel the temperature, the warmth of the blood flow, any air blowing across it, etc. Even though whatever body part you chose was always there, until you put your conscious attention into it, you probably didn't even really notice it.

Get good at this before moving on.

The next version of this is to start to apply this same level of conscious awareness to all of the thoughts and emotional feelings that come up inside of you whenever a strong emotional event takes place in your day to day life. Remember, try as best as you can to just notice these things without judging them as good or bad or trying to fight them. You may not succeed at first and that's ok. It's the practice that we're after.

Once you get a handle on that, you're going to apply it directly to your diet.

Anytime you're making a decision to eat, notice your thoughts and feelings or any sensation whatsoever in your body.

What is prompting you to eat this food? Is it genuine hunger? Is it boredom? Is it a particular thought or feeling? How do you feel when eating? What is it like for you to eat something that is in-line with your desired diet? How does it feel to eat something that isn't a part of your desired diet?

Start to observe this stuff each time you eat, and if it helps, make a journal of your observations.

That's it! It may sound simple, but don't let the simplicity fool you. This exercise **alone** can actually fix unwanted habits overtime, but more importantly it's the foundation of everything else you will do going forward.

Later in this book, we'll cover the absolute best exercise for actually changing your brain to become more focused, aware, and present in every area of your life which will help you become significantly better at practicing daily awareness.

How Can You Completely Change How You Feel About A Diet?

Once you start to gain a greater awareness of what drives your behavior and why you've developed the habits you've developed, you can then start to consciously change your behavior.

I want to make a quick note about the nature of "change." Some people argue they "shouldn't" or don't want to change because they accept themselves as they are. While it's important to accept yourself as you are *now* (as opposed to living in denial), it doesn't mean you can or should remain the exactly as you are now for the rest of your life.

This is true for a couple reasons. One reason is nature dictates that nothing stays exactly the same and therefore everything and everyone **must** change. While an oak tree will always remain *fundamentally* an oak tree, it will also always be either growing or dying and changing with the seasons. It is never the exact same oak tree from one day/moment to the next.

The other more practical reason for wanting to change is that we all have areas of our lives we can improve. That doesn't mean we have to beat ourselves up with where we're at now, it just means living in the present while being future-oriented. It's about accepting both where you're at on the journey of life while accepting the choice that you must *move* forward (therefore change your present location) on that journey.

All in all, you're going to be changing whether you like it or not. You can either choose to be stuck with the habits you've developed over the course of your life through happenstance, or you can choose to take control of your life, actions, and therefore your outcomes. The question is, do you want to leave that change to chance or choice?

This means taking personal responsibility. You may not control everything that happens to you, but you can always control how you *respond* to those things.

This may be some pretty heavy philosophical sort of stuff. I wanted to cover it briefly because, if a person does feel like they *shouldn't* change, then that underlying belief will prevent them from doing the things necessary to change their dietary habits. Since you're reading this book, that obviously means you're the kind of person who wants a better life and is interested in making changes for the better, so I won't keep preaching and philosophizing. Let's get to applying real world tactics to making changes in your life.

Here are four basic ways you can shift your motivation based on your emotional wants:

1. Focus more on the benefits of making the change vs. staying the same

Example with Excitement: A person chooses to focus on the new exciting things they can do when their body is feeling better and how that compensates for less excitement in the foods they're eating. i.e. They become motivated by the prospect of *gaining* pleasure.

2. Focus more on the downside of staying the same vs. changing

Example with Security/Control: A person chooses to focus on the pain that a poor diet would bring them like getting sick and missing out on things they enjoy vs. not having to worry as much about ill health on a better diet. I.E. They become motivated by the prospect of *avoiding* pain.

3. Find an alternative way to satisfy an emotional want

Example with Excitement: A person chooses to play a game instead of eating a desert to add excitement to their life. i.e. They get their emotional needs met through safe and healthy non-dietary means.

Note: This approach can backfire if the substituted behavior isn't healthy. An example of how this would backfire would be someone who instead of smoking starts eating in excess. Or a recovering drug addict resorting to excessive gambling to fulfill their need for excitement.

4. Let go of the emotional attachment or resistance to a behavior.

"Letting go" is a very simple but life changing process. It is essentially the ability we all have to let go of or "release" any feelings, beliefs, attachments, resistances, etc that we have internally. Mastering this technique can give you complete emotional freedom.

Here are some examples of "letting go." A little kid has a fight with his friend, and five minutes later they're playing together like nothing happened. An adult gets cut off in traffic, and five minutes later they've forgotten about it and are chatting with a friend.

But, if these people didn't "let it go," the person who got cut off ends up chasing the other driver down the highway with a bad case of road rage. Or that kid grows up and still broods over that one time Timmy called him a stupid face.

Sometimes people confuse "letting go" with suppressing emotions or "pretending" like nothing is wrong when it's quite the opposite. You instead *welcome* your thoughts and feelings without trying to fight them.

One very simple process of letting go is:

1. **Welcome** all thoughts and feelings without judgment or resistance.

2. Ask yourself, "can I let this go?"

3. Repeat the process of welcoming the thoughts and feelings and asking if you could let it go.

While this is only a basic exercise and there's much more in depth work and explanation that can be done. This one exercise can be a powerful process with practice.

It can be very important to let go of some things because too strong of an attachment to satisfying one's emotional wants can lead to unhealthy addictions or neurotic behavior. If a person has a strong attachment to getting the validation of others, they may engage in all sorts of actions, many of which might not be healthy, to constantly try to get the approval of those around them.

This drive to get validation/approval from others may be part of the reason some people resort to extreme measures of weight loss such as radical diets or even bulimia. The other direction a person may go to is that if they don't get validation from others, that person may *overeat* to compensate for their emotional pain. While the two behaviors may appear to be opposite of one another, they are both driven by an emotional attachment of wanting approval from others.

Note: The actual cause of various eating disorders has a multitude of differing psychological factors. These are just examples to make a point about the influence of seeking validation on human behavior.

It should be pretty obvious that this type of obsessive behavior isn't healthy or desirable. But it doesn't take an actual diagnosed disorder for our emotional wants/needs to be a subtle force in all of our lives leading to unwanted behaviors, addictions, and unhappiness.

So this means learning to "let go" of attachment of wanting other people's validation is necessary not only for happiness, but simply because it would be impossible to always have other people's validation. While I'm using validation as one example, it applies equally to the other emotional wants as it is also impossible to always have complete control over everything, or to always have guaranteed security, or to always be in a state of excitement.

There is nothing wrong with these emotional wants and you can never "get rid" of them as they all serve a useful function. You can also certainly use your understanding of these emotional wants to help get focused on finding motivations for getting yourself to change which we'll do later.

However, I strongly encourage you to recognize that living your life trying to always to satisfy these emotional wants only through *external* means is a surefire way to misery. Rather, a healthier approach is to realize true satisfaction and happiness can only come from *within* yourself.

For more information on "letting go" and emotional management, I highly recommend you read the book "The Sedona

Method" by Hale Dwoskin which is the best resource I've found on the topic. This book alone will likely give you all you need to successfully stick to a diet from an "emotional" point of view in addition to resolving many other emotional issues and addictions a person may have.

The bestselling book The Power Of Now by Eckhart Tolle is another excellent read for understanding acceptance and non-resistance on a deeper level from a more philosophical/spiritual view.

See: http://excuseproof.com/resources/recommended-books

What Is The Common Denominator Among Any Method Of Changing Your Habits?

You'll notice one common theme throughout those four methods of making a change, and that is *focus.* "What you focus on expands" is a powerful truth that is relevant not just for sticking with a diet, but it applies to all areas life.

- Focusing on solutions rather than the problems themselves is the only way to constructively make progress.

- Focusing on the emotions you feel can help you get the message they're trying to tell you vs. repressing them only to have them eat away at you.

- Focusing on the pain of staying the same will prompt you to change for the better.

- Focusing on the benefits of making a positive change will help you enjoy the process.

- Focusing your effort on finding **healthy** means of satisfying wants and desires can help you feel emotionally fulfilled without resorting to unhealthy behaviors.

- Focusing on what you already have and are grateful for can create feelings of abundance in your life so you don't rely on external things (like junk food) to provide that feeling.

- Focusing on your past successes will build your confidence going forward facing new obstacles.

Now that you have a basic understanding of how your emotional wants influence your behavior and that your motivations can be shifted through changing your focus, we can go from the "philosophy" behind all of this and go to the practical application. This means we're going to start applying more exercises to generate motivation *on demand.* This requires actively focusing on the three things you're going to learn about in the next chapter.

Is There A Method That Can Create Unstoppable Motivation?

The "blueprint" to diet success may simply be summed up in this one process:

1. Defining *what it is you don't want* in your life which a poorer diet would create. This could be something like not wanting to be overweight, not wanting to feel run-down, not wanting to prematurely age, not wanting to experience a particular health problem, etc.

2. Defining and *focusing* on *what it is you do want* in your life that a better diet would provide you. This could be a more lean and fit body, more energy, a stronger immune system, freedom from pain and sickness, etc.

3. Determining and *focusing* on *why you want* a better diet in a way that is personal to you. For instance, "so I can feel better" is vague, but "so I can have the energy to play with my kids" is specific and personal.

4. Determining and *focusing* on *how you get* what you want by determining the appropriate actions to take including what behaviors to cease and what behaviors to engage in. This could be eating more vegetables, cutting out excess sugar and junk food, juicing vegetables, learning new recipes, etc.

Quite possibly the biggest reason why people fail to stick with diets is because they don't have good answers to these questions. While most people just assume they know what they want and why they want it, it's very rare to:

Have the right *kind* and *quality* of answers that aligns with one's deepest values and emotional drives.

Sometimes people get really caught up chasing someone else's goals for someone else's reasons instead of truly being clear on what they want and why it really matters to them. You may have experienced this yourself if you've ever reached a goal only to feel empty and unfulfilled despite getting everything you wanted. This is a whole subject unto itself, but I want to point this out so you understand why we're going to be digging as deep as we are in the following chapters which is to prevent this from occurring.

Why Are Some People Unable To "Get" Motivated?

You now know that you must have an answer to these three questions to be motivated towards your desired diet:

A) What do I want?

B) Why do I want it?

C) How will I get it?

But... even though just about everyone can readily give a few answers to these questions, what many people don't know is that it takes a very particular <u>kind</u> of answer to each of these in order for it to "activate" their inner motivation mechanisms.

We're going to cover why most people fall short when it comes to providing accurate answers to these questions, and what you can do to ensure you get very clear and focused so you can set your brain to drive you towards your goals on autopilot.

Defining <u>What</u> You Want

Let's start with the first thing you must do, and that is defining what you want.

Some people will say something like "to be less fat" if focusing on weight loss. Or they'll say "to be healthy" if focused on health.

The reason why these goals are not enough to "activate" their motivation is because they're not clear and specific. What does "less fat" even mean? Losing 1 pound? Losing 20 pounds? Dropping 3 pant sizes? The human mind loves to work towards goals, but those goals must be clearly defined or else it feels like we're wandering aimlessly not quite sure whether or not we're making progress.

Compare "I want to be less fat" to "I want to be a lean 124 lbs with a shapely defined physique that fits into my favorite pair of jeans" or "I want to be a muscular 180 lbs with a ripped six pack and 17 inch biceps that look like mountains."

Compare "I want to be healthy" with "I want to move around pain-free with ease, wake up bursting with energy that lasts throughout the day, and be able to run a mile in under 7 minutes" or "I want to be medication free and have all of my blood parameters at normal levels."

These "whats" are clear and defined, and working towards them is far more rewarding because you'll be able to track and monitor your progress.

Defining <u>Why</u> You Want It

If someone has the desire to "stick to a diet," then there must be something compelling them to want to change from their status quo. These reasons are usually health (more energy, overcoming or preventing disease, etc.) and/or fat loss related, but there can be countless reasons for wanting to change one's diet including ethical and environmental reasons, lifestyle circumstances such as time, and budget, and athletic pursuits.

When I was in high school, I was told my diet was unhealthy by my mom and friends. But that didn't prompt me to change because I didn't know **why** it was unhealthy or how that affected me in my day to day life.

But it was when I learned that my diet was making me weaker and leading me to early aging and disease by causing internal havoc in my body, I realized **why** eating better was important and why I would *benefit* from changing. I saw what I was doing to my body was having *real* negative effects and I wanted to avoid that pain. Before that, eating poorly just didn't mean anything to me personally. So why would I bother to change?

Determining <u>How</u> You'll Get It

While most people think they know what they want and why they want it, it's the "how to get it" type of information that is most in demand and prized.

It's not hard to find a lot of "how-to" advice when it comes to eating better for health, fat loss, or most other goals. But there are a few big problems with this how-to advice.

The first is that there's so much conflicting information out there, people don't know who to trust and what really works. Particularly when how-to information is often combined with hyped up marketing like "how to lose 70 pounds in 7 seconds" type of nonsense. The overwhelming amount of hype out there that people have to try to sort through is one of many reasons I created my blog Excuse Proof Fitness at www.excuseproof.com to get straight to the point of what really works.

The reason you're reading this book is for what I could call the "meta how-to" or the "how-to apply the how-to information." Once you find out what you need to do, then you need to figure out how to actually get yourself to do it! i.e. knowing how to eat for a particular goal and knowing how to *get yourself* to actually eat that way are two different things.

Telling someone to eat a pound of broccoli every week for health and cancer prevention is one thing, but figuring out how one is actually going to prepare that pound of broccoli, make it taste good if they hate it, and then incorporate it into their weekly diet routine is a whole other matter all together.

Oftentimes people are told how to do something, and then are left to simply use willpower to follow through. But willpower alone is *not* the way to achieve long term results. Instead, we're going to set ourselves up for success so that you take action without constant force, and utilize only small amounts of willpower that anyone can muster up in order to making *lasting* change.

How Can You Tap Into Your Deepest Motivational Drives?

Get out a pen and paper or open a blank document on your computer and start writing down the answers to the following questions.

Note: This is something you'll likely come back to again and again, so leave room to revise and add more answers to each of these things.

Step 1:

Write what you *DON'T* want in your life that you believe results from a poor diet.

Is it having or adding excess fat? Is it faster aging and wrinkling? Is it low energy? Is it poor sex drive? Is it disease? Is it an early death and leaving your family behind?

Write down at least one compelling thing you want that is driving you *away* from undesirable eating.

Although I gave broad examples, the more specific and compelling the reasons are for you and your personal circumstances, the better.

Example: "I don't want to have this 23 pounds of excess weight." "I don't want to have these love handles and cellulite." "I don't want to be taking 13 medications and spending $437 a month on medical expenses." Etc.

Step 2:

Write what you DO want in your life that you believe results from a better diet.

Is it a healthier body? Is it more energy and focus? Is it looking better naked? Is it living in line with your ethical beliefs? Is it feeling better about the choices you make? Is it wanting chicks or dudes to dig your six pack?

Write down at least one compelling thing you want that is driving you towards better eating.

Note: You should be able to come up with at least an equal number of things you *do want* by simply providing the opposite of what's on your "*do not want*" list from step 1.

For instance, if someone stated "I don't want to be 20 pounds overweight" in the previous step, they would then say "I want to be 20 pounds lighter (or weigh XYZ pounds) in this step.

Once again, the more specific and personal the better.

Example: "I want to be off all medications." "I want to weigh XYZ pounds and fit into size XYZ clothes." "I want to enjoy clear skin" "I want to live to see my grandchildren graduate college" etc.

A Note On Goal Setting: It's important that your goals seem challenging but obtainable. It's not realistic for a everyone to think they can look like a genetically gifted model or perform like an Olympic athlete. But sometimes we also severely underestimate what we can actually accomplish and never realize what we're truly capable of achieving.

I suggest striving for something that seems a little more than what you're comfortable with, but feel you **can** accomplish.

This is because your goals should be in line with your self-image. In other words, you should be able to visualize your goals and say "I can do that." Even if you don't feel like you can do something *now*, at least you feel you can *learn* and *grow* into being a person who can reach that goal.

Overtime, as you reach higher levels of success, you'll probably realize you're capable of more than you gave yourself credit for and can always aspire to greater and greater things. Remember, it's a never ending journey.

For more on understanding how to improve your self-image for reaching goals and overall happiness, I suggest the book "The New Psycho-Cybernetics" by Maxwell Matlz.

See: http://excuseproof.com/resources/recommended-books

Focus On The Positive: It's important to *recognize* what you don't want, but keep your *focus* only on what you DO want.

Here's why: "*Don't* think of a purple elephant!"

Did you think of one? That's because while the mind is very motivated to avoid painful things (what's found on your "do not want" list), it can't really process "not doing" something without an alternative thing to do instead. Your mind is like a GPS system where instead of putting in all the locations you don't want to go, you must simply put in the one location you *do want* to go to.

So now try this, "instead of thinking of a purple elephant, think of a RED elephant." You'll see it's easier to avoid focusing on a purple elephant if you're given an *alternative* to positively focus on.

This means when it comes to your goals, focus on what you are working towards rather than working away from.

This is actually a big secret to why focusing on *not* eating junk food can actually backfire and simply cause a person to keep thinking about how much they want to eat junk food until they cave into their desire! Instead, one should focus on the alternative thing that they're going to eat or do instead.

Step 3:

Replace the word "want" with the word "choose" anytime you're writing or thinking about your goals.

Example: "I *want* to lose 20 pounds by eating a nutritious diet and making better food choices each day" becomes "I choose to lose 20 pounds by eating a nutritious diet and making better food choices each day."

"I want to take better care of my health" becomes "I choose to take better and better care of my health."

This simple shift in language may seem insignificant, but the implications are huge. This is a very big missing link in most other sources on writing down and thinking about goals.

Try this: change the word "want" to "choose" when stating a goal out loud and notice if you can detect a difference in your body in terms of how you think and feel. Do you feel more empowered? Do you feel more in control? Does the thing you "want" feel more like something that you *can* and *will* have?

What we're going for and that simple shift in feelings has a profound effect in everything you do when pursuing your goals. It also keeps you focused on what you're doing in the <u>present</u> moment rather than getting too caught up in trying to live in the future.

Step 4:

Write any reasons why a poor diet will bring you pain.

A way to determine these reasons are by taking your answer(s) in step 1 (what you don't want), and then exploring how it would make you feel a sense of losing validation, control, security, and/or excitement. Be sure to consider the impact diet has on you both now and in the future, as well as the indirect impact it can have in other areas of your life. Start by using the word "because" and then follow up with your reasons.

For instance: "because a poor diet would rob me of my energy. A lack of energy would keep me from playing with my kids (loss of control) and makes me feel like I'm missing out on what life has to offer (loss of excitement). I'm worried if I kept poor eating habits, it would destroy my health." (loss of security and control)

While you don't necessarily have to link your "reasons why" with the four emotional wants, it can help find more compelling reasons. The biggest mistake people make is they don't know *compelling* and genuine reasons that are personal and "real" to them. Instead they offer generic and vague reasons that sound good, but that don't actually elicit a strong emotional response.

Let's say someone wanted to quit smoking.

Something as simple as: "I want to quit smoking because I don't like that cigarettes unhealthy and have been shown to cause cancer" is not very specific and it's not very personal. It's just not an emotionally powerful enough reason for some people to get motivated enough to change.

You can always dig deeper by asking yourself more and more "why questions." Using the previous example, this person would keep asking why until they get to deeper reasons that eventually really resonate with them.

"Why don't I don't like that cigarettes are unhealthy? Because this can lead to an early death. Why don't I like that they can lead to an early death? Because then I wouldn't be there for my family. Why don't I like that I couldn't be there for my family?"

Now this person is likely starting to tap into some very deep reasons for quitting smoking. Their new "reasons why" could then start to look something like this:

"I want to quick smoking because I couldn't live with the pain of having to explain to my wife that I won't be there for her if I get cancer. I couldn't even imagine having to endure the pain of trying to explain to my kids why I won't see them grow up and graduate college. The heartbreak in their eyes and knowing how I've let people down with my decisions is too much to take. Continuing to smoke could make me feel like I failed to be a good father and provider knowing I can be shortening my life. I love my family more than anything else in this world and I would do anything for their sake. This is the reason I'm **choosing** to be a non-smoker."

Can you imagine the difference in motivation between the first reason why and the later reasons after further exploration?

NOTE: I'm not saying smokers or people who eat a poor diet are bad parents and must change their behaviors. Rather, it's more about illustrating the importance of finding reasons that are **personal** to you and your values. So a family oriented person may wish to link their "reasons why" to how it affects their family, while another person, say someone who runs a business, may link reasons to how their actions affect their business and so on. Whatever reasons you come up with must be your own and resonate with you and your values.

Step 5:

Write any reasons why you gain pleasure from a better diet.

A way to determine these reasons are by taking your answer(s) in step 2 (what you do want), and then exploring how it would make you feel a greater sense of validation, control, security, and/or excitement. Use the same suggestions in the previous step for this step.

For instance: "because a great diet fills me with energy and vitality. Having more energy allows me to be more productive at work (in control of my life) and makes me feel like I'm really enjoying some of the best things life has to offer (more excitement). I know following this better diet will enhance my health allowing me to live longer (more security and control). Better diet choices keep me looking young and fit (more validation).

Tips On Finding Reasons Why To Avoid A Poor Diet And Eat A Better Diet:

Try to find reasons that relate to your core values. Look at what you're already passionate about and do effortlessly. How do you spend most of your time? If you had all the time and money in the world, what would you do with your life? (If you haven't considered these things, then perhaps some soul searching is the first step.) Ask yourself what it is about those things that drives you and excites you.

When you find the underlying values and reasons why you do what you do, connect those back to how those things will be affected for the worse by an undesirable diet and affected for the better by a beneficial diet.

So if you really value freedom, explore how poor diet choices will limit your freedom in life and better diet choices will give you more freedom to do what you love. For some it could be hiking, playing sports, or just enjoying everyday activities more.

It's also important to find things that are **inherently** enjoyable about eating a better diet. Eating well for some far off reward (like losing weight) can be motivating, but not as motivating as eating better because of what it brings you right **NOW**.

A classic case of this with a non-diet example would be kids playing sports for the fun of it. They love every moment of it because it's a game. But as soon as they start getting pressured to perform better and win (focus on the outcome rather than the process), things like practicing transition from "fun" to "work."

That's not to say there's anything wrong with external motivators like winning, or in the case of a diet losing weight as an example. But the difference between a diet being "work" or a way of life has a lot to do with whether you focus **more** on the external rewards that come later or more on the instrinsic benefits you find during the process itself. For myself, eating well is enjoyable and rewarding for its own sake regardless of what happens months down the road, therefore sticking with it is far easier.

Some benefits I focus on when eating healthy are the energy I get from eating healthy foods, the confidence I feel knowing I make good choices about how I take care of my body, and the fun of trying new healthy recipes.

If you're still struggling for personal reasons why to stick with a diet, consider that:

The food you put into your body not only affects the way your body looks, but also influences the very thoughts you think and feelings you have. Your diet plays a role in either feeling dull and lifeless, or feeling alive and full of energy and vitality. The aches and pains in the body can be aggravated or relieved by dietary measures. The very success of your relationships, business or job, memory, brain health, and everything else is influenced on some level (obviously not completely) by your diet.

All in all, there is no separating any other area of life from the foods you eat or vice-versa. Everything is connected.

Also, educating yourself about about the pros and cons of certain diets and ways of eating is a great way to remind yourself why you want to make better choices with your diet.

There are many great books, blogs, dvds, youtube videos, etc for educating yourself. But as a warning, I also encourage you to not get too caught up with any style of diet as "dogma." Researching too much can actually just lead to confusion as there is so much conflicting information out there.

Here are some useful resources to educate yourself why eating healthy is beneficial:

www.mercola.com – The most popular alternative health blog. His newsletter is a good source of tips for improving health and avoiding disease.

www.renegadehealth.com – Kevin Gianni runs one of my favorite blogs for getting "non-dogmatic" view on healthy eating through diet, with a bit of a vegetarian slant. Kevin draws from numerous resources and is a super likeable guy. Definitely worth subscribing to his newsletter for tons of information on not only what you can do to improve health, but learn why certain foods may be better for health and others damaging. He also has good recipes and guest posts frequently posted.

www.thebestdayever.com/news/podcast - The Best Day Ever podcast is a treasure trove of cutting edge health, anti-aging/longevity, and disease prevention information. David Wolfe is one of the most popular figures in the health community.

www.bewellbuzz.com – Be Well Buzz and The Be Well Buzz podcast (www.bewellbuzz.com/category/podcast), run by nutritionist Shawn Stevenson from www.theshawnstevensonmodel.com/ provide not only great tips and tricks for healthy living, but go really in depth scientific detail that everyday people can understand as to why these things are important.

www.alanaragon.com – Alan's work is more suited to the fitness and bodybuilding community. He's by far one of the most well known experts for being able to take complex scientific studies and distill the information for the educated masses who want to use diet and supplementation to look and feel better. He dispels a lot of myths in the fitness community.

Fat, Sick, and Nearly Dead – A documentary on the effects of a poor diet and how they can be reversed through healthier habits like vegetable juicing. Watch for free on Hulu at: www.hulu.com/watch/289122

Note: Even though I recommend these as useful diet resources sources, it doesn't mean I believe everything they put out or that they're the best for you. I also know some people out there will argue the credibility of these sources (saying such and such person is a "quack") which would be unavoidable regardless of what resources I recommend. The key is to continually educate yourself from a variety of sources and find what works for you. Please try not to get too caught up into which expert is "right" and which one is "wrong" because you'll never find anyone right 100% of the time.

Step 6:

Write down how to take action to adjust your diet to reach your goals.

Since this book is about how to get yourself to stick to a diet, I'm assuming you either know what kind of diet you want to eat, or are resourceful enough to track that information down.

But it's ok if you're not exactly sure at this point about what you need to do or how to get started. The key is to start doing *anything* you know can and should be doing. Or alternatively, start tracking that information down.

Sample things you could include on your action plan:

1. Complete the exercises this book

2. Learn one new healthy recipe to make this week

3. Throw out the junk food in my kitchen

4. Buy some healthy snacks I can keep in my car or at work

5. Replace sugary drinks with water

These actions are unique to you, your circumstances, and your desired diet.

Some people for instance may already be successful in following their desired diet, but they just want to make their diet *easier* to follow and not something they do by constant "force." So for them they may include more educational things like learning new recipes and studying health resources to remind them of why they follow their diet.

Stop reading here until you've completed all six steps.

If you've got them done, great! Congratulations for doing far more than most people ever do to ensure they get what they want.

If you *haven't* completed these steps yet, then ask yourself why you're reading a book that's giving you the tools to change your life and not even applying the information. Go back and make sure these exercises are complete, even if it's only a single answer. Remember, you can always come back and add more later.

Ok great! Now you've gotten an overall idea of <u>what</u> you want, <u>why</u> you want it, and <u>how</u> you can start taking action reach your goals. For some people, just getting clear on this is all they need to stick to a diet.

But we're just getting started. Now we can dive right into the *daily* action steps needed to stick to a diet. This will include some of the most powerful exercises out there to really make sure you stick with your diet even if you're faced with tasty temptations, challenging circumstances, and wavering willpower.

When Can Goals Actually Be Detrimental To Achieving Success?

While I strongly recommend having goals to begin with, it's also important that goals are kept in their proper context. Otherwise, goals and being too obsessed with "not being there yet" can actually sabotage a person from getting results! Or even worse, a person can end up completely miserable even if they *do* reach their goals.

Let's use weight loss as an example because it's easy to measure.

If a person wants to lose 30 pounds in 3 months, but it ends up taking them 6 months, did not reaching that particular goal really matter in the long run? Or if a person does reach their goal and loses 30 pounds in 3 months, but gains all that weight back in 6 months, did reaching that goal really matter?

The potential problem with goals is not so much goals in themselves. Rather, it's in the way people approach goals.

One unfortunate thing that can happen is a person sets a goal, let's say to follow a particular diet for 3 months and lose 30 pounds. They hate the diet, but they force themselves to follow their exact diet plan for 3 months until they finally reach their desired goal.

What might they do at this point? Well now that they've reached their goal, they don't need that stupid horrible diet anymore, right? So they drop the diet and "celebrate" with their favorite comfort foods they've been depriving themselves of all that time. They let themselves go, and even if not right away, within a year or two they've gained all the weight back and then some.

Or alternatively, they keep "forcing" themselves to eat a certain way even though they're not happy, stressed out, and are miserable. They haven't really made that diet part of their natural lifestyle, rather they just follow the diet recommendations out of fear that any deviation will cause them to lose what they've worked so hard for.

So if a person can't break a diet without risking losing their results, and if they can't follow a diet without feeling stressed out, what can they do?

The best way to resolve this is to simply approach healthy eating as a lifestyle, not a set of rules to live by every meal of everyday. This usually means a certain degree of flexibility and striving for 80-90% compliance rather than obsessing over every dietary detail.

This also means that goals are NOT the end, but rather they're themselves a *means* to an end. That end is developing better **habits**, behaviors, and strategies for balancing healthy eating with the other important areas of your life.

Once a person has developed the right habits, things no longer need to be "forced." Therefore, the best way to "stick" with a particular diet is to make following that diet a habit. It becomes integrated with your life so you no longer have to think about it.

It would literally be harder for me to eat fast food and junk food than eat my typical healthier diet. My taste buds now enjoy nutritious whole foods. I know how to eat more economically making my own food so it would actually cost more money to eat fast food or junk food. It would also take me more time and effort to drive to a fast food place and pick up a meal than cooking something myself. (You'll find out some of my fast cooking secrets later on)

Another reason you want to strive for habits is because you can "cheat" on occasion and it won't necessarily hurt anything. This means you can be at ease knowing you still get to enjoy the great foods out there without feeling overly deprived.

I can eat junk food on occasion, go out with friends to a nice restaurant and order whatever I want, and treat myself to some sugary dessert for a celebration. Because it's so rare for me to engage in these behaviors, and because my "default" setting is to eat well and exercise hard, "cheating" on occasion has little to no consequences.

What you have is not a result of simply everything you do, but more the result of everything you do *consistently*.

I should note that way I developed those strong habits was by having strict goals and plans that I followed for weeks, months, and even years on end before diverging from them. Once the desired behaviors became consistent, only then could I stray away and not fear falling off track.

This may sound difficult, but with a systematic plan in place like you're getting in this book, it can be done with relative ease. It's like the saying/riddle, "How can you eat an elephant? One bite at a time."

For an excellent article on living productively without goals, check out Leo Babauta's article on his site Zen Habits at http://zenhabits.net/no-goal

How Can You Change Any Long Standing Habits Permanently?

The way we're going to do this is through a "30 day challenge." The idea here is to pick one or a couple new dietary habits that you'd like to change. This can either be a behavior you want to eliminate, a behavior you want to incorporate, or ideally a substitution of one "bad" habit for an alternative "better" habit.

Create and write down a "30 Day Challenge" identifying one habit you would like to change that will move you closer to your ideal diet.

Include **what** you're doing, **why** you're doing it, and **how** you're going to do it.

For instance: "(*what*) I'm replacing all sugary soft drinks with water (*why*) because soft drinks are causing me to gain excess fat and (*how*) I'm going to do it by carrying a large 1 gallon container of water with me at all times throughout my day so I'm never without water. (*how*) I will add some fresh lemon to the water and a bit of stevia if I'm looking to enhance the flavor."

or

"(*what*) I will learn a new recipe every week (*why*) because if I enjoy the taste of the food I eat, I will easily be able to stick with my diet. (*why*) My biggest challenge is that I hate "health" foods and don't have much time to prepare my own food, but I also know there are some really tasty meals that only take a few minutes to prepare. (*why*) So learning these new recipes will really help me stick to my diet. (*how*) I will subscribe to at least 3 recipe blogs and youtube channels, and once a week I will browse through them for 15 minutes until I find a recipe that looks good. (*how*) I will set aside 30 minutes on Sunday afternoon from 3:30-4:00pm to make that week's recipe.

Read your 30 day challenge goal to yourself daily to keep your focus on it.

Visualize yourself doing the actions, enjoying the process, and succeeding.

The 30 day challenge will be something that is challenging (duh!) but easy enough you know you'll be able to succeed. After 30 days, choose a new "30 day challenge" while still, as best as possible, *maintaining* your previous habit you developed the 30 days prior. Each month, you're building upon what you've done before until your day to day habits have become completely transformed.

If you feel you can do something more significant, like take on changing multiple habits, or making more significant changes to your diet all at once, then go for it. But this must be based on all the other things you have going on in your life. A lot of times, we get really gung-ho at first only to burn out later. This is exactly what we're trying to prevent. So it's better to error on the side of doing just enough at first and adding more over time vs. overdoing it at first and burning out quickly.

So ask yourself, what things can I do for the next thirty days I know I'll succeed at, but still be able to continue with for all the following months once I start adding more stuff in?

The idea here is that you'll only need to focus on a few things a month so you're not getting overwhelmed. This prevents the typical problem of people trying to completely change all of their dietary habits all at once, and then quickly burning out and getting overwhelmed.

Why Do People Screw Up If They Try To Use Willpower Alone?

Up to this point in the book I've been making it a point to clarify that willpower *alone* is not the answer to sticking to a diet. But, that doesn't mean you won't need *any* willpower. In fact, without willpower, you will absolutely fail to make any successful change in your life.

To read this book, do the exercises, and even change what your mind is focusing on all requires an act of the will. The reason why willpower doesn't work by *itself* is because very few things we do are purely acts of the will, but rather acts of habit.

The simplest way to look at willpower that I've found is that it is what is needed to set the ball rolling, but habits are what keeps the ball rolling in motion with relative ease. Or, willpower is the force used to launch a rocket into space, but once it's in space it stays in motion from the previous force that was generated.

Think about how much effort (will) it takes to first learn how to drive a car. A person requires complete focus and attention and it is likely a bit challenging at first. But then when that person has made driving a normal routine (part of their brain's programming) they can easily carry on a conversation or flip through the radio stations while driving without any major effort.

The good news is if you're following the simple practice of focusing on only modifying one or a few habits each month, and these changes are reasonable, that *should* be well within your willpower's capabilities.

But, some people still struggle to muster up the will to make better choices no matter how insignificant they are. What they don't realize is they may be robbing themselves of their willpower without even knowing it! There is a *very* important thing research has shown must be managed or else it will sabotage any attempt you make to change. Read the next chapter to discover how to overcome limited willpower and succeed.

What Is The #1 Hidden Cause Of Bad Habits, Failures, and Disease?

There is something even worse than junk food when it comes to destroying health. This thing has been linked having a role in over 90% of chronic diseases. It can actually alter the genetic expression of an individual meaning that health and weight issues stemming from genetic "problems" may actually be influenced (for better or worse) by this. Studies have shown too much exposure to this is likely the reason why people fail to make better dietary choices no matter how internally "motivated" they are.

To make matters even worse, almost *everyone* these days is <u>severely</u> affected by it.

What is it?

It's *too much* **stress**! While most people have a general idea that "stress is bad," very few people realize just how many things stress impacts and to what degree. The recent research showing the damaging effects of stress, combined with the research on how many people are enduring unnaturally high level of stress in our modern world, has lead me and numerous experts to realize getting a handle on stress should be a bigger priority than just about anything else someone can do for their health and well-being.

Before going further, I should note the caveat here is *too much* stress. A little bit of stress is not only acceptable, but actually beneficial. Exercise is a form of stress that when done in appropriate amounts, the body responds to by growing stronger and more resilient. But too much exercise can cause injury and breakdown meaning there is a balance that must be achieved.

This is true for other forms of stress as well (psychological and physiological), so the key thing here is not to worry about "getting rid" of all stress (or getting stressed out about stress), but rather learning how to *manage* stress so it actually makes you stronger instead of tearing you down.

Besides the direct impact excess stress has on the health of the body, it's the indirect effects we are most concerned with here. Research and real world experience has shown that the more stress one endures, the less "willpower" they have. In fact, those who've experienced a lot of stress actually have areas of their brain shrunk down which are responsible for decision making and self-control. See: http://www.ncbi.nlm.nih.gov/pubmed/22218286

Many other studies have shown the negative effects stress has in other areas of the brain as well. Too much stress can actually make it harder for the brain to handle stress! So it creates a downward spiral of stress – bad decisions – more stress – more bad decisions – inability to handle stress – stress becomes out of control – developing chronic disease – etc.

Stress is the reason why it can be so hard to make a change in your life, even if that change is a positive one you *want* to make. That's because *any* change in your habits can elicit some degree of a stress response. A *small* stress response is actually important because it tells the brain to lay down new neural pathways associated with learning. This stress response tells the brain "this is important so pay attention."

The problem is that when a person *already* has too much stress in their lives from everything else they have going on, any attempt to make a change, such as making better food choices, will add to the <u>overall</u> stress burden they're experiencing. The brain and body will do everything to resist adding that further stress because it knows that all this stress is, quite literally, "poisoning" the body. In other words, too much stress makes it *very difficult* to make changes to your habits. Your body's built in defense mechanisms will fight to keep you from adding further stress to your life until you get a handle on any excess stress you're experiencing.

There are three ways we can get around this.

● The first way, which I consider essential, is to reduce overall stress in your life. Unless you're a zen monk, you probably are experiencing more stress (at least in certain areas of life) than you'd like. While our ancestors needed a stress response to fight or flight from "real" danger, our modern world often creates a type of chronic psychological stress the human body/mind was never designed to handle.

● The second way, which is incorporated into this book through the 30 Day Challenge, is to only take on a few changes in your life *at a time*. This reduces the amount of stress you're adding to your body when choosing to make better habits for yourself.

● The third way, which I provide exercises for later on, is to shift your "psychology" surrounding stressful situations so you can handle them without your body creating as much of a stress response.

What One Practice Has The Most Power To Transform Your Life?

We know too much stress shrinks your brain, but what if there is actually a way to *grow* your brain, *alter* your genetics (epigenetics), and make you become more resilient and impervious to stress?

Meditation is the "Yin" to stress' "Yang." In addition to thousands of years of successful use, there are now a crap-ton of scientific studies showing the benefits of meditation for reducing stress as well as altering the brain, genes, and behavior. Here are just a few interesting articles:

http://www.sciencedaily.com/releases/2012/06/120613183813.htm

http://www.sciencedaily.com/releases/2012/03/120314170647.htm

http://www.plosone.org/article/info:doi/10.1371/journal.pone.0002576

http://www.mindful.org/news/meditation-leads-to-better-decision-making

http://www.frontiersin.org/decision_neuroscience/10.3389/fnins.2011.00049/abstract

While I could cite many more studies to confirm all of this, let's just get straight to how to mediate for all of these benefits.

The simplest meditation is a breathing mindfulness meditation where you:

- Sit in a relaxed upright position with your spine straight and feet flat on the floor. Alternatively, if you're comfortable in a seated meditation position you may do that.

- Start to <u>focus</u> on your breathing in and out. You may choose to consciously slow your breathing rate.

- If it helps you relax, you can mentally "scan" your body head to toe relaxing each muscle and body part.

- Continue this for 1-15 minutes (start with just a few minutes daily), or as long as comfortable.

- As you get more proficient in being able to focus only on your breath during meditation, you may begin to simply observe your thoughts coming and going. Rather than "fight" any thoughts, simply watch them occur and pass through your awareness. It can help to think of yourself not as "me" or "my thoughts," but as an overall awareness of those things.

- While the purpose of meditation isn't necessarily to try to stop thoughts but rather "observe" them, if you really want to quiet your mind, you may mentally make the effort to "watch for" the next thought that is going to occur. Ironically, the more you try to watch for the next thought to arise, the less thoughts seem to come until your mind becomes quiet and still.

Even though meditation is an *active* process, don't worry about "screwing it up" and remember as long as you do it regularly with focused intent, even if your mind wanders a lot at first, you'll start to get better.

This practice can and will change your life in ways you may have never imagined with regular use. This isn't just some overly esoteric spiritual "woo woo" if that's not your thing. It's confirmed science with thousands of years of real world success.

Here are some more resources from Zen Habits on how to meditate and make it part of your life:

www.zenhabits.net/meditate

http://zenhabits.net/meditation-for-beginners-20-practical-tips-for-quieting-the-mind

www.zenhabits.net/build-strength

How Are Some People Destroying Their Health And Willpower Without Even Knowing It?

Want to know a great way to torture people, deprive them of their willpower, and get them to do or tell you anything you want them to?

Well... hopefully you don't. But knowing what the single most effective way of sucking a person's willpower dry is could be useful information if you **don't** want to fall victim to it. Unfortunately, many people are doing this practice *to themselves* without even realizing it.

You can do all of the motivation exercises in the world, but if you're not getting enough sleep, it's going to impair some very important areas of the brain responsible for decision making. In fact, studies have shown a direct impact that lack of sleep has on making poor food choices.

http://healthland.time.com/2012/06/11/why-sleepy-people-reach-for-junk-food

Granted, we could go on forever on how poor sleep promotes faster aging, reduced immune system response, and is responsible for a significant amounts of accidents and fatalities in car crashes, work deaths, etc. But, since this about sticking to a diet, let's just keep in mind that prioritizing your sleep should be as high as prioritizing what foods you eat.

So now that you know why you benefit from getting enough sleep, let's look at how you can enhance your sleep and make sure you can easily fall *and stay* asleep.

1. Reduce exposure to artificial light and stimulating things like computers and TVs before bed. Dim bedroom lights if possible. Wear a sleeping mask if needed. Make sure windows are covered to prevent excess sun exposure or light exposure if an issue in the mornings. Reading or

meditation is a good way to wind down.

2. Make sure you have adequate magnesium levels. Magnesium deficiency is extremely common and a typical reason for insomnia. Magnesium oil or 500 mg of chelated magnesium (like magnesium citrate) is recommended. To test mineral levels, see www.spectracell.com.

3. Getting "grounded," also called "earthing," has been shown to normalize cortisol levels and circadian rhythms. Grounding is also associated with significant pain reduction and less inflammation. It is quite possibly the "missing link" to good health. See the book Earthing by Clinton Ober and Steven Sinatra (www.excuseproof.com/resources and earthinginstitute.net) Inexpensive grounding mats may be purchased to sleep at http:/www.earthing.com/Shop_s/1824.htm. I suggest simply purchasing the Universal Mat, using it while on the computer and sleeping on it at bedtime which is what I do.

4. Some herbs like Valerian, Passion Flower, and Chamomile help to calm the nerves and relax. Try making one of these herbal teas or take a high quality herbal sleep aid if you need a natural way to wind down.

What Technique Is Essential To Avoid Feeling Overwhelmed?

If there's one common denominator among stressed out people in our modern world, it's the feeling that there's just too much stuff to do and not enough time. It's not uncommon to be so busy that the thought of adding one more burden, like figuring out new foods to eat, is just too much. Sometimes just thinking of changing a diet seems like it would be filled with so much stuff to figure out and do, it's a lot easier to just not even bother and hit up a local fast food place instead.

What I'm about to share with you is not only extremely effective for sticking with a diet, but it has been responsible for helping many people find the joy of a "less-stress" life. The difference before and after practicing this technique is night and day in terms of how overwhelmed I feel (which isn't to say I still don't get overwhelmed at times, I just now know how to handle it).

The easiest way to sum up this technique is this: **Prioritize**

Prioritizing isn't just about figuring out what you need to do, but it's just as importantly about figuring out what you *don't* need to do.

Staring at a never-ending "to-do list" is stressful for even the most driven and hard working among us. But looking at a list with only a few key "must get done" activities or overall projects to be completed for the day is far easier. The shorter you can make your "to-do list", or as we'll call it "priority list," for each day the better.

To do this, take an accurate assessment of your life and current goals. Then before going to bed or first thing in the morning, write down the top 1-5 things that need to get done and take care of those things. Ideally, knock those things out before doing anything else lower on your priority list. Of course, things related to your diet and 30 day challenge will be on that priority list.

Figuring out what the biggest priorities are to you is something you'll need to do on your own. But since this is about reducing stress, I can give you some great tips to figure out what you *don't* need to be doing each day:

1. Ask yourself how much "busy" work you do that might *feel* productive, but really isn't. Shuffling papers, checking emails, long phone conversations, solving other people's problems, etc. Ask yourself "is this really the most important thing to be doing right now?" Also ask, "can I hire or get someone else to do this busy work for me, or can I be ok not doing it at all?"

2. It's very tempting to want to work on things that *are* priorities in our lives, but are not priorities just *right now.* For instance, when writing this book and I was doing research, I focused my attention on doing research each day. If there was something else relevant to writing this book I was thinking about or caught myself doing such figuring out the design for the cover, I would catch myself in the moment and simply write a note to address it later. If I found a cover design I liked, I'd make a note about it but then I'd get right back to work. My favorite way of doing this is by keeping notes on my computer (I sometimes incorporate www.evernote.com and www.simpleology.com) to get all of my thoughts that I need to remember stored away. This keeps me focused on what is most *immediately* important without diverting my attention (creating stress) to all sorts of other things that can be taken care of later that day, week, month, or even years down the road.

3. Multitasking is only effective for certain types of activities; those that don't require much conscious focus. Things like cleaning while listening to an audio book or talking on the phone while taking a walk. Remember to focus your attention on whatever you're doing in that moment 100%, and for other things going through your mind, remind yourself you can always cross that bridge when you get there.

4. Focus on changing only a few areas of your life at a time in order to "stretch" your comfort zone rather than break it. A New Year's Resolution to completely change one's diet and

start exercising 5 times a week won't work for most busy and stressed out people because it's too much all at once, but making a few gradual changes each month will ensure success.

5. Reduce the options you have when making choices. Research has shown that when we're given **too many** choices, it reduces the likelihood of making **any** choice. This is actually a benefit of some diets for certain people because having less choices of what to eat actually makes it easier (less stressful) to decide what to eat. Remember, more isn't always better, so "keep it simple stupid."

How Can A Few Words Curb Cravings And Keep You From Giving Into Temptations?

Language is incredibly powerful. The very words you use in your day to day language, both spoken out loud and in your head, affect the very way you think and feel.

Earlier in this book, I gave you a simple "mind hack" that showed you how you can take the phrase "I want" and change it to "I choose" to instantly feel more empowered and "present."

Now I'm going to show you a few other "tricks" that can instantly change your feelings and mindset just by substituting a few words in your vocabulary when making day to day decisions.

Language Hack #1: "I can't" and "I have to" becomes "I choose to."

An LA Times article mentioned simply changing the phrase "I can't" (restrictive) to "I don't" (choice) improves dietary compliance and cuts cravings. http://www.latimes.com/health/la-he-cravings-20120721,0,7652489.story

A reason for this is probably because we as human beings naturally sometimes rebel against anything that will limit our freedom (called reactance in psychology), and as you can now see, this comes from the core emotional wanting to be in control. Those who fail to stick to a diet, because of control issues, likely feel that the restriction and deprivation of a diet plan makes them feel trapped and enslaved to the dictations of that plan.

Just imagine someone telling you that "you can't do that" or "you're not allowed to do that" and see how that makes you feel. While some people will have more or less issues with "threats" to their sense of freedom (some people prefer to be controlled rather than be in control), the point is that if you find you want to rebel against limitation, you'll need to know how to work with this.

Those that successfully stick to a diet, even a restrictive one, often feel on some level their diet makes them *more* in control. The idea that they control their food intake by choice rather than by cravings makes them feel in control.

I prefer the word "choose" rather than "don't" because it keeps your mind focused on the positive intent. It also reminds you that you are always in control, and you're *choosing* to engage in different behaviors because you've *chosen* something **better** for yourself and your body. It also reminds you that you "can" have something else if you want, but then you must accept responsibility for your actions.

Examples: Instead of "I can't eat this doughnut," try saying "I choose to keep my body healthy by only feeding it healthy foods" or "I choose to eat an apple instead."

Instead of "I have to eat this salad," try saying "I choose to eat this salad."

Want to make "I choose to" even more powerful?

Follow up the phrase with the word "because" to remind yourself *why* you're making that choice and keep yourself feeling positive and motivated rather than deprived. "I choose to avoid the doughnut <u>because</u> it will slow down my progress" "I choose to eat an apple <u>because</u> it will give me the leaner healthier body I really want." "I choose to eat a salad <u>because</u> it nourishes my body and keeps me full of energy."

Language Hack #2: "Would I Rather..."

This is my favorite "back pocket" way to deal with any cravings, addictions, or temptations. If you get nothing else out of this book, write down this phrase and apply it every time you're struggling with a temptation.

The exercise is simply to ask yourself a question that starts with "would I rather..." and then insert the undesired behavior and undesired consequence followed by the positive behavior and positive consequence.

"Would I rather eat these cookies and stay overweight forever and feeling guilty **OR** eat this apple and have a lean fit body that people admire feeling proud of myself and happy?"

"Would I rather go out with friends and pig out only to feel like crap and regret my decision OR stick to my diet plan and feel great about myself and earn the respect of my friends as they see my perseverance?"

Of course, we can all recognize that eating cookies on occasion won't really keep someone overweight forever, but the point is to illustrate that you're always making trade-offs with any behavior you engage in. So find what is real and meaningful to you, and use "would I rather" to reinforce that your choices will bring about consequences for better or worse.

TIP: A variation of this is something I've found to be one of the most powerful ways to rid myself personally of obsessive thoughts. It is asking: "Do I want this to have power over me or would I rather be free?"

An example with obsessing over a junk food I crave. "Do I want this food to have power over me, or would I rather be free?"

Let's say someone has made me angry. I ask myself "Do I want to let this person have power over me to make me feel angry, or would I rather be free?"

If I keep thinking about something I want to do later: "Do I want these thoughts and obsessions to have power over me, or would I rather be free?"

Thoughts and feelings that were driving me crazy have completely vanished never to return after asking myself a question like this. Sometimes it takes a bit of really focusing on the question, but it works. The reasons this works is slightly complicated, and may have something to do with my personality highly valuing autonomy and freedom. But I feel it is important to include it in here so you can see how questions can be used to shift your mindset and feelings about things.

Language Hack #3: The "Excuse Eliminator"

All of these "language hacks" have something in common, and

that is they are in the form of a question. Questions are a powerful way to access your subconscious mind.

When someone tells you something, or you tell yourself something, your mind can either accept or reject it. But asking a question always demands your mind tries to come up with an answer. (You probably noticed I made every chapter title in this book a question.)

You can use this principle of question asking to your advantage in ways that are so powerful, it can transform every single area of you life.

One of the reasons why questions work is because you come up with your own answers vs. some other person telling you what you "should" do. To overcome excuses and start finding answers, replace a "dis-empowering declaration" with an "empowering question."

● Not enough time? Instead of saying "I don't have time," you may ask yourself "What can I do with the time I have?" "What is a faster way of doing things" "When will I have the time?" "Can I stop doing some of the things that are eating up my time?"

● Not enough money? Instead of saying "I don't have enough money," you may ask yourself "What can I do with the money I have?" "How can I make more money?" "Are there other things I can do that don't require as much money?"

● Feeling unmotivated? Instead of saying "I don't feel like it," you may ask yourself "How can I make this more exciting?" "Why do I *want* to do it?" "Could I just let myself try it?" "Can I just do the first step and see where I go from there?"

● Feeling stressed out? Instead of saying "I'm stressed out" you may ask yourself, "What is the **one** thing I can focus on doing right now?" "Can I allow myself to relax and let go of some of this stress?" "Can I see everything that is right within this present moment?"

- Feeling miserable? Instead of saying "My life sucks," you may ask yourself "What am I grateful for?"

All of these various "language hacks" require regular use to make them habits and therefore truly effective. They can have "instant" effects. These techniques are like a musical instrument that you practice daily and they become natural in terms of how you speak and think. It's also like a musical instrument in that it's not so much the words you say that will make as much of a difference as it is the feelings and intent you put into those words and questions.

What Force Is Stronger Than Willpower?

The spiritual guru Yogananda has a saying that "environment is stronger than will-power."

We are influenced to a strong degree by our environment. This is because we have something built into our biology called called "mirror neurons." Mirror neurons literally recreate, in our minds, what we experience externally with our senses. These mirror neurons may be why seeing someone yawn can make you yawn. Or hearing others laugh can make you want to laugh (even if you don't know what they're laughing about).

This is an incredibly useful part of our biology as it is a built-in mechanism for both greater connection with one another as well as improved learning. A baby learns to walk and talk from seeing and hearing others walk and talk. The transition from observing to doing takes the ability to "mirror" what we take in from our environment.

This doesn't change into adulthood. While we may develop greater cognitive abilities to think through our actions, that doesn't mean our thoughts, beliefs, and behaviors are completely independent of the environment we're in. If you have ever hung around a certain person for a while and noticed yourself starting to talk like them. This would be firsthand experience of how this mechanism works.

What this means for sticking with a diet, or any other habit for that matter, is that your environment may have more to do with success than your willpower.

But the good news is, you can use your willpower to *set up* your environment for success.

How can one's environment be detrimental to dieting success?

Here are just a few common examples:

1. Having a kitchen stocked full of foods that you wish to avoid.

2. Eating out at places that will put tempting foods in front of you.

3. Sharing your goals and accomplishments with people who will criticize you or not support you.

4. Hanging out with others who don't share similar goals and ambitions.

None of these things are *inherently* bad.

It would be impossible to always avoid tempting foods. It would also be particularly difficult to always avoid people who won't support you, especially when they are family, co-workers, and close friends.

But the idea here is that you'll want to be aware of these things having an influence, and either minimize your exposure to them, and/or compensate with more positive influences in your environment.

What are some practical tips for dealing with "negative" environments?

If you feel a person won't support your decision to take better care of yourself and follow a diet, ask yourself if you really need to share it with them. There's nothing wrong with keeping goals between you and only those that will support you. There's not even anything wrong with keeping goals to yourself as research has shown that, despite all the recommendations to share your goals, sometimes sharing them can actually make you less likely to achieve them. (We'll cover when you should share your goals)

While others may have your best interest in mind, anytime someone sees someone else making a decision to change their life for the better, it can remind them of how they are falling short of their own potential. This means that even if you decide to eat a better diet for your health and well-being, some people may criticize you for it, even the ones closet to you.

If this happens, realize that it is *their* own issues and has nothing to do with you. While this will likely be unavoidable, you can certainly minimize this occurrence by only sharing your goals and aspirations with those you know will be a supportive and helpful force.

You may find yourself in a situation where others are questioning you about the foods you're eating. Rather than get caught up in arguments or wasting your time trying to explain it, sometimes it's better to just let them know you've decided to take better care of yourself and leave it at that. If you feel like they're pressuring you emotionally to not stick with a diet, you can simply ask yourself "do they have the results I want?" If not, why even bother listening to them?

Some research has in fact shown sharing your goals can make you **less** likely to achieve them. While this is the exact opposite of what is sometimes recommended, we're going to tread carefully by only sharing your goals in a particular way for a certain purpose. Keeping goals a "secret" can actually be quite powerful.

Control your environment consciously by removing unhealthy foods, and even "unhealthy people" whenever possible.

Clean out your kitchen from any junk that doesn't need to be there. If you have a family, ask for their support and do your best to get them on board and explain the reasons why this is important to you.

If you have friends, co-workers, family members, acquaintances, or anyone else that tends to bring you down either with regards to diet or any other area of life, ask yourself "do I really need to be spending as much time with these people?"

The idea isn't to be cold-hearted and disregard them completely, but out of respect for your own well-being, sometimes exposure to certain people needs to be reduced or cut off completely.

This isn't just an issue with regards to your diet, it can be a manner of others constantly complaining to you about their problems and draining your energy and mood. This stress can have a negative effect on *every* area of your life, and therefore indirectly affect your dieting success. While they may mean no harm, it can be best to explain to these people that while you love them and value your relationship with them, the topic of conversations must change if you wish to stay in close contact.

What are some common ways one's environment could be helpful to dieting success?

There are many ways to set up your environment for success, here are a few:

1. Hanging out with peers whom you aspire to be like

2. Having a mentor or a coach who keeps you accountable

3. Having the right kinds of foods in your kitchen

4. Visual cues like inspirational posters

5. Reading books and stories about people you admire

6. Reading, listening to, or watching educational material on why diet is important and how to improve your diet

7. Engaging in visualization to see and feel your goals as a reality

In the end, there are always going to be environmental factors that can potentially help or hurt us. We can't get rid of everything "bad" in our environment no matter how much we try, and that's ok. Sometimes "negative" things are needed to make us stronger. But for now, realize that taking a few steps to manage your environment can save you tremendous amounts of stress and difficulty down the road.

In the following chapters, we're going to cover how to use an external influence that research has shown may be the single most important thing you can use to guarantee you stick with a diet.

What Is The #1 Way To Guarantee You Stick To Your Diet?

Why will an ordinary person push themselves to the limits of what the human body is capable of when they enter a military boot camp? Why will some work tirelessly at a job they hate even though they can't seem to muster up the willpower to take up a hobby they've always wanted to try? What do the world's most successful and hard working people, like Olympic athletes, CEOs, or stay-at-home moms all have in common?

Accountability

All of these scenarios entail a person who are accountable for their actions.

A soldier in training not only has to answer to their drill sergeant, but their fellow soldiers both in training and combat whom are depending on them to get the job done.

A person will work harder if they have a boss to answer to or a family depending on them to pay the bills.

A stay-at-home mom will sacrifice everything for the sake of her kids who are depending on her to meet their needs.

But who holds you accountable if you want to start eating better? If you mess up your diet, are there any consequences?

For some people a lack of external accountability with their diet is why they fail time and time again.

While self-accountability is something great to strive for, if environment is stronger than willpower, then the best way to use your environment to ensure success is to have someone or something keep you accountable for your actions.

How To Create Accountability

1. Get an "accountability partner." This can be a friend, mentor, or anyone else who will support you in your 30 day challenge and overall goal. The people keeping you

accountable are the only people you really need to share your goals, endeavours, fears, and successes with.

2. Journal about your successes and failures frequently, including how well you've been sticking with your "30 day challenge."

3. Check in with your accountability partner at least once or twice a week and share your successes and failures. If you have any failures, rather than provide excuses, provide the ways you can prevent it from happening again if possible. While you don't need to let them in on everything, you should make sure they keep you accountable to the most challenging things for you get done.

4. If need be, set up a system of rewards and punishments for successes or failure. Rewards should ideally be something unrelated to diet. Punishments should be things that are healthy and that you would benefit from doing anyways. (Run a mile, clean up your place, etc.)

5. If you'd like to create further accountability, you can create a free blog (www.wordpress.com or www.blogger.com) and share your results and journal online. Track down others and follow their work, and have them follow yours. If you really enjoy helping others, see your experience eating better as a means of sharing tips, tricks, and struggles with others so you can be a source of help and inspiration. This is particularly useful for people who are highly motivated by helping others.

6. You should only share your goals with your friends and those closest to you **if** they will support you and question your progress to keep you on track. You may share your results on the Excuse Proof Fitness facebook page at www.facebook.com/excuseproof to further spread the word and get support.

Can You "Brainwash" Yourself To Stick To A Diet?

One of the biggest challenges people have when trying to "get motivated" is listening to others why one should eat better. Unless the reasons you have are **your own**, you'll always feel like you're doing things because you "should" rather than because you "want to."

The following exercise is quite possibly the most powerful one in this entire book because it has the power to tap into your deepest belief systems and create change from the inside out.

Here are the steps to the process:

1. Find your highest values - The simplest way to do this is to consider what you love most in life and your passions. What do you do effortlessly? What would you give anything for? Then ask yourself "what is the underlying value that drives this behavior?" There are some tests and lists that can help spur ideas (www.listofvalues.com), but you can simply come up with your own words to describe what your values are.

2. Write a hand written essay arguing why sticking to a diet will align with your values, and why not sticking to a diet will go against your values

3. Stand in front of a mirror and read your essay aloud to yourself. Do this with conviction, really selling your own beliefs to yourself.

4. Publicly share your values essay with your accountability partner, and ideally as many supportive people as possible - Post it online to a blog, journal, as a facebook note, etc.

Example:

Let's say someone values freedom very highly. This person will want to include reasons why sticking with a diet allows them more freedom, to the point that eating well is *essential* for freedom. They will also explain how eating a poor diet will cost them their freedom.

"Eating a poor diet robs me of my health, vitality, and energy leaving them feeling weak and helpless. It's only through taking care of one's body through a good diet that they can experience the most freedom from disease and sickness, freedom to move freely, and freedom from the slavery of food addictions. By cooking my own meals, I have freedom to eat whatever I feel like and not rely on prepackaged food or other people for my meals. Eating a poor diet would make me feel lethargic and unable to do the things I want to do." Etc.

Then, after covering as many points on this value, one can move to another value like contribution.

"Eating well is necessary in order to bring my best self to serve others. If I eat a poor diet, I'm sick and tired more often and won't be there to help others as well as I could. People are depending on me, and I will let them down if my poor diet robs me of my health, energy, and upbeat spirit. Eating well is necessary to ensure I live a longer and healthier life to be there for my family." Etc.

When you create YOUR argument based on YOUR truth and in alignment with YOUR values, you'll be reprogramming your own mindset to succeed not based on what others tell you you "should" want, but based on how a diet works with your own inner values.

The way this really works is through publicly sharing. We may be able to write one thing but do another, but it's very difficult to publicly state something to other people and then go back on our word. By creating an essay that *you* truly believe in, and then sharing it with others, you will start convincing yourself each day of the truth of what you wrote until it becomes your belief system on a very deep level. And for reasons beyond the scope of this book, the act of seeing yourself in a mirror works to create a degree of accountability even if others are not present.

Warning: While this exercise is safe, be careful about taking specific dietary beliefs to the *extreme*. So be mindful that you're establishing healthy diet beliefs that support your values rather than getting too dogmatic about "right" and "wrong" foods and diets.

How Can You Finally Overcome Sugar, Salt, And Food Cravings?

While some cravings may disappear over time as your taste buds adjust to a new style of eating, sometimes cravings are physiological rather than psychological.

Here are some tips for dealing with cravings for sweets and sugar.

Sweet cravings can be a symptom of an imbalance in the gut microflora (gut bacteria). Taking a clove of raw garlic chopped up in half a cup of water each morning can help kill off some of the harmful bacteria and yeast.

Also be sure to include some cultured food in your diet like cultured vegetables (raw sauerkraut, raw kimchi, kefir, homemade yogurt, etc.) and/or take a quality probiotic supplement to get more beneficial bacteria in the gut. This is helpful not only for sugar cravings, but immunity, skin and hair appearance, and overall health.

Note: There is a difference in the effect of different probiotic strains and supplements. You may need to try a variety to see what gives you best results.

See: excuseproof.com/probiotics

Resources and starter cultures for culturing your own vegetables and kefir: http://bodyecology.com

Try stevia or xylitol in place of sugar as sweeteners. I generally recommend avoiding most other artificial sweeteners like aspartame (equal) and sucralose (splenda). Some artificial sweeteners have been associated with interfering with hunger mechanisms and linked to weight gain.

Moderate amounts of good quality honey and blackstrap molasses are better alternatives to refined sugar because they are full of beneficial minerals. Studies show honey doesn't affect triglyercides like pure fructose and table sugar. Molasses is rich in chromium which helps regulate blood sugar balance. That being said, if you're sensitive to sugar, still practice moderation with these.

Mineral deficiencies may promote sugar cravings. You can get tested with a blood test to find any particular deficiencies. See www.spectracell.com for details. I recommend using whole food sources to correct deficiencies before utilizing supplements.

High stress and excess cortisol can fuel sugar cravings. Besides practicing the stress reduction techniques in this book, one of the most effective and affordable herbs for aiding in stress reduction and balancing cortisol is Ashwagandha. The Sensoril extract has been scientifically shown to bring cortisol levels back to or near normal levels very effectively.

For more details, see: http://excuseproof.com/favorite-supplements/

Taking a teaspoon of apple cider vinegar with water at meal times will not only enhance digestion and improve health, but the sour flavor can offset sugar cravings. Another option is to add some fresh lemon juice to water. These are both great healthy habits to use regardless of whether or not they help with sugar cravings.

Here are some simple tips to address salt cravings:

Rather than excessively restrict salt, use a quality unrefined salt like a Himalyan salt, Celtic sea salt, Redmond salt, Wright Salt, or other mineral rich salt. Salt cravings may be mineral/electrolyte cravings stemming from deficiency and an unrefined salt will provide additional minerals. You can make your own healthy salty rich snack like kale chips using an unrefined salt to get the added minerals including the potassium in kale.

How To Make Kale Chips – excuseproof.com/kalechips

Eat mineral and nutrient rich whole food supplements like spirulina, chlorella, and sea based vegetables like kelp and dulse.

Test for mineral imbalances. See www.spectracell.com for details.

Here are some tips for dealing with hunger cravings:

1. Fill up on fiber rich vegetables like leafy greens, celery, and beans that fill you up.

2. Green tea and yerba matte teas are healthy drinks with moderate amounts of caffeine which can help curb appetite.

3. Caralluma is a safe and effective supplement (it's an edible cactus) for reducing appetite. It has shown to increase energy and safely promoting fat loss while. See: http://excuseproof.com/favorite-supplements

How Can "Not Having Time" Be A Lie?

There is no such thing as "not having enough time" because we don't "have" or "own" time. The old saying "we all have 24 hours in a day" is true no matter how busy our lives are. What we do have is the *choice* as to what we're going to do in a 24 hour period of a day.

You're not managing time, you're managing the **activities** that last a period of time.

So "I don't have enough time for that" would more accurately be stated "that's not a big enough priority for me right now."

Since I'm all about practicality, let's look at some ways you can cut down on wasting your time by focusing on what you *can* control, and that is the choice as to how you spend "your" time.

1. If there are activities that don't require a lot of focus, you may multitask. Preparing food while talking with a friend for instance.

2. Cook in bulk all at once. In under 5 minutes, I can prepare food for up to 2-3 days by using a slow-cooker (aka crock-pot). I simply put the ingredients in, let it cook overnight or during the day, and come back to several days worth of healthy food.

For more information on cooking in bulk, see these videos:

excuseproof.com/fastmeals

excuseproof.com/fastchili

If you want some free slow-cooker recipes, check out this website:

www.allfreeslowcookerrecipes.com/

Learn recipes that are super fast. Many great recipes only take 5-10 minutes to make, and when you make a lot at once, that means you can prepare all of your meals in under an hour a week.

Here are some free resources for healthy recipes:

youtube.com/leanbodylifestyle which is now switching over to youtube.com/michaelkoryfitness

www.youtube.com/excuseproof

http://www.bodybuilding.com/fun/bbmainnut.htm

You can even take one day a week to cook everything, and then store each meal in separate storage containers (I like locking to-go containers). You can either keep the meals frozen and thaw the night before and/or store the meals in the refrigerator.

Utilize time saving kitchen devices. Small blenders, hand choppers, juicers, and slow-cookers are all relatively inexpensive, but they can far make up for their modest cost with the time they save.

A Magic Bullet Blender or a similar compact blender is quite possibly one of the best investments you can ever make. I use it to create tons of sauces and smoothies. Clean up is easy, and I can store the containers in the refrigerator with my sauces inside which I prepare in bulk.

The next book I will be releasing is specially designed for eating healthy in a hurry with tips, tricks, and recipes I use to eat healthy no matter how crazy my schedule is. If you'd like more time saving strategies, visit www.excuseproof.com and sign up for the free newsletter to get my Survival Guide with some of my best time saving tips!

How Can "Health Food" Taste Amazing?

Besides simply learning better recipes that are in line with your diet (a subject of a future book of mine), there are a few simple substitutions you can make when preparing food and cooking that can be healthier options. Particularly for people who aren't trying to follow a very strict diet, but just want to reduce their overall calories, avoid allergies, and/or make healthier food choices.

Here are some of my favorite alternatives to traditional ingredients:

1. You can replace vegetable oils in baking recipes with an equal amount of applesauce. Coconut oil also makes a good alternative.

2. Wheat in baked goods can be replaced (or cut down) with almond flour, buckwheat flour, rice flour, coconut flour (in small amounts), and various gluten-free flours.

3. Pasta wheat noodles can be replaced with quinoa noodles, rice noodles, buckwheat noodles, and sliced zucchini.

4. Milk (lactose) can be replaced with almond milk, boxed coconut milk, hemp milk, or oat milk. For those with digestive issues, kefir and yogurt may be better tolerated as they are often virtually lactose free.

5. Sour cream in some recipes can be replaced with greek yogurt or canned coconut milk.

6. Refined sugar can be replaced with stevia (calorie free), xylitol (less calories), coconut sugar, blackstrap molasses, honey, and lakanto (calorie free).

7. Homemade sauces can be used in place of store bought condiments to spice up foods and enhance the health value. Sauces made in a small blender often only take a few seconds to prepare and can be easily stored in the refrigerator for up to a week.

Here are some simple sauce ideas:

1. Store bought salsa blended with fresh avocado for instant guacamole.

2. 1 cup fresh or frozen mango, 1 cup fresh tomato, 1 or 2 Tbs. balsamic vinegar, Two mandarin oranges (optional) blended for a tasty salad dressing.

3. 1 cup Greek yogurt, 2 tbsp. Italian seasoning, two cloves of garlic, and dijon mustard if desired blended for a tangy dip or dressing.

4. Lemon juice, apple cider vinegar, and cayenne pepper for a spicy salad dressing.

Additional sauce recipes:

http://www.cookinglight.com/food/quick-healthy/six-simple-sauce-recipes-00400000048440/

http://greekfood.about.com/od/dipsspreadspures1/r/Tzatziki.htm

http://www.foodnetwork.com/recipes/alton-brown/horseradish-cream-sauce-recipe/index.html

How Can You Stick To A Diet On A Budget?

1. Local farmer's markets often have high quality food produced without pesticides (organic quality) at a much lower price than in the grocery store.

To find local food sources and farmer's markets, visit

www.eatwellguide.org

2. If shopping for organic food, prioritize the most important foods to buy organic. These are the foods with the highest pesticide levels like apples, strawberries, and potatoes. Some foods like bananas and avocados aren't as important to buy organic from a pesticide standpoint due to their thick skins. For a list of the highest and lowest pesticide levels on produce, visit: www.ewg.org/foodnews/summary/

Meats and dairy tend to accumulate toxins so they're better foods to purchase organic or from a local farmer that raises the animals under good conditions. Grass-fed beef has a healthier fat profile than traditional corn-fed beef.

Corn and soy are often genetically modified and best purchased organic.

http://www.healthychild.org/live-healthy/checklist/top_ten_genetically_engineered_food_crops/

3. Local co-ops will let you get food directly from a farm at a hefty discount, often purchased in bulk. To find a local co-op in your area, visit localharvest.org. This is one of my favorite methods of getting the highest quality foods at the lowest prices, as well as supporting local farmers and cutting down on the environmental impact of transporting food.

4. Purchase food in bulk either through online stores or bulk food stores. A great online bulk food store is barryfarm.com. Even expensive health food stores often have a bulk food section where you can find very good deals.

5. Many grocery stores have special prices on food about to expire, particularly meats. Shop for the bargains and then find creative ways to prepare whatever you end up with.

Where Can I Get Discount Protein Shakes?

Supplements and protein shakes are one thing that many people spend a fortune on and they don't need to. If you know where to look, you can purchase whatever kind of protein (whey, hemp, casein, rice, egg, etc.) online, custom mix different types of protein, add your own ingredients, flavoring, sweeteners, etc, and all at wholesale prices.

My favorite place to get affordable protein shakes is True Nutrition (formerly True Protein) at www.truenutrition.com. Look for the "raw ingredients" and "custom mix" tabs at the top left.

You may use my discount code DKD714 save even more on your order.

I usually order my protein from True Nutrition as they have the highest quality sources, best prices, and the ability to custom make your own blend to match whatever tastes and diet you have.

Another good source of discount protein is www.proteinfactory.com which is similar to True Nutrition.

A typical pound of low quality whey protein at a retail store may cost anywhere from $20-$30. A "designer" (aka hyped up overpriced) whey protein can be upwards of $50 a pound. You can find the same or better quality whey for on True Nutrition for $7-$12 a pound.

Their deals on vegan proteins like hemp, pea, and rice are excellent alternatives to the very high priced vegan proteins at health food stores as well.

Where Can I Get Discount Supplements?

For discounts on supplements, the most consistently affordable prices with the widest selection is iHerb.com.

Use code hec508 to save $5 (or $10 on orders over $40) on your first order at iHerb .

Amazon.com now has a wide variety of nutritional supplements at very competitive prices. With free shipping on many products with purchases over $25, this is often a good choice.

Swanson vitamins at www.swansonvitamins.com offers very high quality supplements at much more affordable prices than other companies that typically mark up their prices to pay for expensive marketing campaigns.

Where Can I Get Affordable Fat Loss and Muscle Gain Supplements in Bulk?

Besides True Nutrition and iHerb, www.nutraplanet.com is an excellent resource for fat loss and muscle gain supplements at a very low price. They offer a very large selection of bulk ingredients for those who like to mix their own supplements and save some money.

Finally, www.bodybuilding.com offers a large variety of fat loss and muscle gain products with a price match option to match competitor's prices.

What If You Don't Know Anything About Cooking?

1. The transition from eating out a lot, or making prepackaged foods may be eased with healthy canned foods. Canned beans, canned fish, and canned soups helped me a lot when I first got started until I learned to make them myself from fresh ingredients. I still use them in a pinch and they can be more affordable.

2. Learn "idiot-proof" recipes at first like salads, stir fried vegetables, soups, stews, chili, smoothies, juices, etc.

3. Even if you eat out, you can still find a variety of options at restaurants to fit just about any diet. The biggest hidden things to watch out for are the ingredients in sauces and condiments as well as cooking oils.

To find healthy dining options in your area, see www.healthydiningfinder.com/

What About The Strict Rules That Make Diets So Difficult?

The key thing to remember is the best diet is the one you can actually stick to. While striving for 100% compliance to a particular way of eating can be useful, more often finding a realistic balance between "ideal" and "practical" can mean better results in the long run with both your body and sanity.

Here are a couple common things that are, in my humble opinion, **myths** about what constitutes healthy eating.

Myth 1: "You must eat a large breakfast" – The research on diet and intermittent fasting shows that not only is a large breakfast not necessary so long as your overall calories remain under control throughout the day.

If you enjoy a large breakfast and you feel fine eating one, great. Go for it!

But if eating a large breakfast or any breakfast for that matter doesn't jive with your lifestyle or body, then don't feel like you "have to" eat one because that's the typical "dogma" in our culture. The most important thing is that you eat the appropriate amount of calories by the end of the day. The timing doesn't matter as much as some people think.

Myth 2: "You must eat 4-6 small meals a day to lose weight or build muscle" – Once again, not necessarily a scientific "fact." If it works for you then you can go with it. But like breakfast, do your own research before coming to the conclusion it is something you "must" do in order to lose weight

See: http://www.leangains.com/2010/10/top-ten-fasting-myths-debunked.html for more research and information from Martin Berkin on breakfast and frequent meals affecting health and body composition.

I will note that women seem to respond better to more frequent small meals while men seem to handle intermittent fasting approaches better. This is of course just a general observation.

Myth 3: "You must do this 100% to see results" - This is more common in the slightly "extreme" diet groups. Since the purpose of this book is not to tell you how to eat, I would simply suggest taking things like "you must eat 100% raw," "you must eat 100% plant food," "you must avoid grains 100%," "you must avoid sugar 100%," and the like with a seriously big grain of salt. It's unlikely there is one "best" diet, and if there is, good luck sifting and sorting through all the conflicting experts trying to find who has discover it.

It may be possible that for short periods of time, 100% acceptance or avoidance of certain foods or eating styles can be important, but rarely when looking at long-term eating habits will anything need to be so "all-or-nothing."

In my years of studying nutrition, I was surprised to find out many people preaching "extreme" diets often fail to follow those diets themselves. Or at least not for long periods of time.

Blood tests are one of the most accurate ways to diagnose what is or isn't working for you rather than blindly following any one guru.

On a more general note, allowing yourself some breathing room, whether that's by eating a small portion of some of your favorite foods each day or a few times a week can go a long way towards keeping your sanity. There are very few foods out there so terrible that a small amount will have major long term consequences.

That being said, if you find yourself "addicted" to certain foods and can't enjoy only a *small* portion, those foods are best avoided all together. If you can prove to yourself you don't really **need** that food to be happy by going a long period without it, you'll often outgrow any addictive desire for it. Eventually, you can probably add it back into your diet and find you can enjoy it in small quantities without needing to go overboard.

For instance, I used to be "addicted" to peanut butter. But after going without it for a few months, I find I can now take it or leave it.

While there are different opinions as to whether it's better to allow yourself to have your favorite treats on occasion to remain "sane" or avoid them all together, I actually prefer the latter UNTIL a person has broken any addictions. The reason being is that, I think there is something powerful about freeing yourself from feeling like you "have to" have anything in particular. If you're happiness is dependent on the food you eat, that may be a sign of deeper issues to work through.

Since this isn't a book on spiritualism and the virtues of non-attachment, I'll simply let you decide for yourself what is most appropriate.

What Is The One Approach Almost Everyone Agrees Improves Health?

In all of my years of research, I have found nothing more profound and well agreed upon for improving health, fat loss, muscle gain, and various blood test parameters as much as fasting.

Thousands of years of use and testimonials to its benefits are hard to beat. And the research on prolonging life span has found calorie restriction to be the most effective means for "shutting off" aging genes and "turning on" youthful healthy genes.

In theory, fasting shouldn't conflict with most diets.

The simplest approach for fasting is to go on a 24 hour fast once or twice a week. An example would be eating dinner at 6pm, and then not eating anything else until 6pm the following night.

However, plenty of water should still be consumed during any fast.

Longer fasts may be done for up to 3 days on either water or fresh vegetable juice for those in good health. Extremely long fasts should be done under supervision of a qualified professional.

What Are The Best Dietary "Tricks" To Enhance Fat Loss?

I believe fat loss is best achieved as a matter of lifestyle and eating well vs. using "tricks" for short term results. The reason being is that if someone achieves fat loss, but isn't able to sustain their new weight through regular healthy lifestyle habits, it defeats the purpose. Long term extremely restrictive diets have been shown to shut down the metabolism and make it far harder to have a fit body for the long-term.

There are a few diet "tricks" to enhance the fat loss process. I want to make a caveat that these are not *necessary* approaches, and they may *not* be for everyone.

The first "trick" is intermittent fasting. There are two approaches to this:

1. Fast for 16 hours a day and eat within an 8 hour period. This is commonly called the Lean Gains approach as it was popularized by Martin Berkhan of www.leangains.com and it is what I typically follow most days myself.

2. The second approach I recommend involves fasting for a 24 hour period once or twice a week. It was popularized in the fitness community by Brad Pilon who has an ebook entitled Eat Stop Eat. www.eatstopeat.com

For more information on fasting approaches, see this great article by Mark from www.marksdailyapple.com here: www.marksdailyapple.com/why-fast-part-six-choosing-a-method/

The other "trick" is to utilize cheat days or "reload" days. Cheat days are days where you allow yourself to eat whatever you want, ideally in the form of additional carbohydrates, and perhaps as much as you want after a period of dietary restriction. These work on both a physiological level and psychological level.

Physiologically, they prevent metabolic "shut-down" or hitting a plateau in weight loss from prolonged calorie restriction. You may have heard that eating too little will shut down your metabolism, and this can be avoided by having a cheat day once every week or two.

It also works psychologically because it's easier to stick with a more strict way of eating if you know you will be able to "let lose" and eat whatever you want on occasion.

I must warn this can work against you if you decide to indulge in addicting foods before you've developed healthier eating habits. I highly suggest making eating well a way of life and habitual before delving into a more advanced approach like this, but regardless of what you decide to do it will be effective.

A way to "supercharge" this technique is to have a cheat day, and follow it up with a fast day. The two extremes work to really amp up fat loss while balancing out the calorie intake between the two days. This is an advanced strategy, and it works incredibly well for fast fat loss.

What If I Screw Things Up?

Falling down is part of the process of learning to walk, and so is getting back up. When you were a baby, you didn't let failure stop you. It's only after we become conditioned as adults that we let the myth of failure keep us from the life we truly want.

The only way a dietary mess up will actually hurt you in the long run is if you fail to get back on track. Only a foolish person says "I messed up my diet today so I might as well just eat whatever I want for the rest of the week or just give up all together." This is the easy way out.

But you're stronger and smarter than that. You know that a failure isn't the end of the road, but the opportunity to learn how to become greater than you were when you made that mistake.

Failures can be "successful learning experiences." In fact, "failing" provides some of the most valuable lessons you can ever get. Likewise, success can lead some people to get complacent and stop trying.

All great people have failed many more times than they succeeded. This is how they *became* great.

Watch and inspirational video on how all great achievers fail before they succeed here: excuseproof.com/famousfailures

You must rekindle that fire that was in you as a child to learn and grow no matter how many bumps and bruises you get along the way. If you don't make mistakes, you're not playing the game.

Nothing you can read in this book or hear from others will have as profound of an impact as what you directly experience yourself be it a success or failure. While gaining the wisdom of others is valuable, the wisdom gained from your own experience is far more "tangible."

While the only way you can truly fail is to quit, recognize that even then quitting has its place. So long as you quit on the "details" but stay committed the destination, you're still on track for success.

For instance, if you're goal is better health, and a certain dietary approach isn't working for you no matter what you do, then perhaps you should quit! It would actually be insanely stupid to keep going along with stubborn persistence if what you're doing isn't working and expecting it to magically get different results.

If a detail of your plan doesn't work, or the plan itself isn't working, then quit and **replace** them with something else. While you may have to take a detour if a certain path is closed down, that's no reason to just pack up and go home. So keep your eye on the goal, embrace failures and roadblocks as inevitable, and don't forget the best part is not reaching your destination, but the ride along the way.

Finally, instead of always dwelling on failures, be sure to celebrate your successes. Do this with your accountability partner, and enjoy feeling good about how far you've come. While there's a fine line between celebrating successes and getting too complacent, it all comes down to enjoying the process. The more you can enjoy the simple process of changing yourself for the better each day without being too focused on the daily ups and downs, the more successful and **happier** you will be.

In fact, the biggest reason I'm so passionate about health and fitness is because I enjoy the process of constant self improvement without getting too caught up in any particular outcome. It may take you time to find this balance, but letting go of outcome dependency and focusing on the process is ultimately the way to achieve the balance and freedom in life we all ultimately desire.

Can You Summarize The Basics Of How To Stick To A Diet?

Checklist:

1. I have established **what** I want my diet to be like and **what** benefits I wish to receive.

2. I have established **why** I'm improving my diet and how my motivations align with **my** values.

3. I have determined **how** I am going to improve my diet with specific action steps, and how I will stay motivated with on-going education.

4. I have set up a 30-day challenge to eliminate an undesirable habit and/or add in a more beneficial dietary habit.

5. I continuously focus myself on my reasons *why* I'm making each dietary choice I make. I remind myself that I'm in control by saying "I choose this because" and asking "would I rather..." when making daily dietary decisions.

6. I have a means of accountability, including a partner that I check in with at least once a week.

7. I recognize how *not* sticking to a diet will negatively affect my body, life, and overall goals. If I feel it's appropriate, I know the external "punishments" (safe and beneficial things like exercise, cleaning, skipping a tv show, paying an accountability partner money, etc) for not following through.

8. I also clearly recognize the rewards of sticking to a diet both with the benefits to my body, health, and overall life as well as any potential "rewards" I've set up for myself for success.

9. I continually strengthen my overall motivations with ongoing education and by asking myself what my goals are, why they're important, and how I'm going to achieve them.

This doesn't have to be hard or time-consuming, it could simply be following a few health newsletters here and there reading a book every now and then. Picking up a new recipes, healthy tips, etc. to make the process more enjoyable.

10. I focus on the process rather than the goal. I recognize this is a lifestyle, and therefore developing habits that work with my life rather than against it are of the up most importance. If I make mistakes, and I will at times, I get up and keep going and enjoy the opportunity I have to learn from them.

11. I have fun and don't get too caught up in "obsessing" about my diet and health. I remember that letting go of stress and enjoying myself just as I am now is the best thing I can ever do for my health and happiness.

Where Do You Go From Here?

Looking for more health and fitness tips:

Besides the resources I've provided in this book, you'll want to check out my free blog, youtube channel, and newsletter with more tips and tricks at:

- excuseproof.com

- www.youtube.com/excuseproof

- www.twitter.com/excuseproof

- www.facebook.com/excuseproof

Looking for a specific exercise and diet program for fat loss, health, and/or muscle gain?

There's a lot of hyped up products out there when it comes to diets and exercise programs promising to get people to burn fat and get a "six pack." That being said, there are a few courses I can highly recommend.

My most strongly recommended body transformation program is LGN365 by fitness trainer and author JC Deen of www.jcdfitness.com

I had the honor of contributing to this course because I believe in JC's work and the results he gets so much. Read my review of it here:
http://excuseproof.com/lgn365review

I also love Dave Ruel's cookbooks. He has both muscle building and fat burning cookbooks, although realistically you can pretty much use either one for each goal and adjust the serving sizes accordingly. You can find out more at these links:

Fat Loss Recipes:

http://excuseproof.com/fatloss-cookbook

Muscle Gain Recipes:

http://excuseproof.com/muscle-cookbook

Congratulations!

You've made it through the book, great job! You've already shown your commitment to learn. But remember, true knowledge is applied knowledge. So get out here and make use of this life changing information. If you have any questions, please contact me at info@excuseproof.com and I will be glad to assist.

If you enjoyed this book, please write a review!

If you enjoyed this book, it would mean a lot to me if you would please take a moment to write an honest review on Amazon by visiting excuseproof.com/diet or http://www.amazon.com/How-Stick-Diet-Unstoppable-ebook/dp/B009GQ4E4W and sharing what you learned and how it has helped you because that help others just like you learn how they can get the same results by purchasing this book. I strongly believe that this information will help change people's lives, and you can help too by sharing your experiences with others. I will be extremely grateful and so will the people that you help inspire to take control of their health. Thank you!

Made in the USA
Middletown, DE
11 November 2020